Jim Pollard is a freelance  was editor of *Arthritis Ne* recently Director of Communications for the voluntary organisation Arthritis Care. He has a repetitive strain injury.

Jacky Fleming is a best-selling cartoonist. Her books, *Be a Bloody Train Driver*, *Never Give Up*, *Falling in Love*, and *Dear Katie* are published by Penguin.

GETTING A GRIP

*Self help for arthritis
and rheumatism*

Jim Pollard

HEADLINE

Copyright © 1996 Jim Pollard
Cartoons Copyright © 1996 Jacky Fleming

The right of Jim Pollard to be identified as the Author of the Work has been asserted by him in accordance with the Copyright, Designs and Patents Act 1988.

First published in 1996
by HEADLINE BOOK PUBLISHING

10 9 8 7 6 5 4 3 2 1

All rights reserved. No part of this publication may be reproduced, stored in a retrieval system, or transmitted, in any form or by any means, without the prior written permission of the publisher, nor be otherwise circulated in any form of binding or cover other than that in which it is published and without a similar condition being imposed on the subsequent purchaser.

ISBN 0 7472 5360 9

Typeset by
Letterpart Limited, Reigate, Surrey

Printed and bound in Great Britain by
Cox & Wyman Ltd, Reading, Berks

HEADLINE BOOK PUBLISHING
A division of Hodder Headline PLC
338 Euston Road
London NW1 3BH

This book is dedicated to the memory of
Frances Coles and Mark Dodds

Contents

1. Introduction   1

2. Types of Arthritis   5
   *Osteoarthritis, Rheumatoid arthritis, Back pain,
   Ankylosing spondylitis, Gout, Systemic lupus
   erythematosus, Reactive arthritis, Psoriatic arthritis,
   Arthritis in children, Muscular manifestations,
   Osteoporosis, Sjogren's syndrome, Work-related
   arthritis/RSI, Other types of arthritis,
   Is arthritis hereditary?*

3. How Do You Feel?   25

4. Arthritis and the Health Professionals   37
   *General practitioners, Hospital consultants,
   Physiotherapists, Occupational therapists,
   Hospital surgeons, Community Care,
   Getting the best out of your health professionals*

5. Arthritis and Drugs   51
   *Analgesics, NSAIDS, DMARDS,
   Anti-malarial drugs, Immunosuppressors,
   Steroids, How to get the best out of drugs*

6. Arthritis and Complementary Therapies   65
   *How to choose a therapist, Acupuncture,
   Alexander Technique, Chiropractic, Herbal medicine,*

Homeopathy, Massage and aromatherapy, Osteopathy, Reflexology, Yoga

7. Arthritis and Diet   89
   What is a healthy diet?, Diet and arthritis

8. Arthritis and the Mind   103
   Self-image, Your arthritis is your business, Self-management, Pain, Stress, Relaxation, Meditation, Counselling and psychotherapy, Personal development, Self-help groups

9. Arthritis and the Body   121
   Stretching exercises, Strengthening exercises, Endurance exercise, Everyday exercise

10. Arthritis and Others   131
    Only you understand, Building self-esteem, Communication, Making love

11. Arthritis at Home and Work   139
    What things are difficult for you?, Arthritis at home, Arthritis at work, Social Security benefits, The wider environment, Out and about

12. Your Way Ahead   161

13. The Arthritis Directory   163
    Bibliography, Addresses

    Index   175

Acknowledgements

A very big thank you to all the people with arthritis and the many former colleagues who have shared their stories and helped in the preparation of this book. Some names have been changed.

I am also extremely grateful to Arthritis Care for permission to quote from their publications and I would like to acknowledge my debt in particular to Olivia Hanscombe for much of the information on the immune system on pages 53–4, from Arthritis Care's special magazine, *The Balanced Approach*; Dr Gail Darlington for her comments on pages 97–8, from Arthritis Care's magazine, *Food for Thought*; and to Penny Boot (a.k.a. Kata Kolbert) for *Our Relationships, Our Sexuality*. The diagram of the joint on page 6 is © Head Design Ltd. Many thanks, also, to Kate Lorig, for permission to quote from her *Arthritis Helpbook* on pages 140–2, and to Cathy Irving, Susy Chaplin and John Heyderman for their assistance with the Arthritis Directory.

CHAPTER 1

Introduction

Do you have pains in your joints? Fingers, elbows, shoulders, hips, knees, ankles, feet? Perhaps it comes and goes. It may be accompanied by swelling, tiredness and/or flu-like symptoms? Or was it triggered by a sports injury, an over-enthusiastic sliding tackle or an unintentional ski-jump? Perhaps it first appeared accompanied by something else? An infection or psoriasis? Did you just wake up with it one day or did it come on gradually over time?

Doctors see dozens of people with these symptoms every day. It has been estimated that one in every four appointments with a local family doctor, or GP, will concern what we generally refer to as arthritis or rheumatism. If you have these symptoms, you've probably seen a doctor already. If you haven't seen one, it would be worth making an appointment.

If you have arthritis you are in good company. From pop stars and actors to members of the Royal family, from captains of industry to captains of cricket teams, there's a lot of it about. Perhaps eight million people in the UK have arthritis to a significant degree.

For some people it can be very severe. It may require the use of a wheelchair or operations to replace damaged hips or knee joints. For the vast majority it is not like this. I hope the ideas in this book will be useful to anyone with arthritis, however severe or mild.

Your arthritis may not be severe, but that does not mean that it is not serious. Far from it. However, the fact that it is so common often means that arthritis is seen as trivial. We all know an aunt, an uncle, a grandparent or even a pet cat or dog with arthritis. Mention to anyone that you've got it and they'll tell you all about who they know that has it, probably at length. Throw in the jokes that arthritis inevitably attracts because of its inaccurate association with ageing, and it's no wonder that we tend to keep quiet about our own experiences of it.

The problem is complicated by the fact that it is so difficult to define. For a start, there are perhaps as many as two hundred types of arthritis. Put simply, arthritis involves inflammation of, disease of, or damage to the joints of the body. All types of arthritis involve a joint or joints in some way. The main symptoms are pain and loss of mobility. The difficulty in coming up with a clear definition contributes to the general view of it as a trivial condition.

For many readers, arthritis may be simply a matter of the occasional visit to the GP. Or, if you've encountered one of the less-enlightened members of the medical profession, perhaps only the one visit. There are doctors (amongst others) who will tell you that you'll 'just have to live with it', that 'it's just wear and tear, what do you expect at your age?' or that 'there's not much you can do about it'. These attitudes are wrong. The truth is that there is a lot you can do, and much you can ask your doctors to help you with.

So, let's correct some of the common myths about arthritis.

First, it is not the inevitable result of ageing. It affects people of all ages and from all sections of the community. Certainly osteoarthritis, the most common form, tends to affect you more as you get older, but to see this as the result of ageing is over-simplistic. It can affect anyone of any age at any time. In this country, there are over one million people with arthritis under the age of forty-five, including 15,000 children. There are a further two and a half to three million of working age, and perhaps four million over sixty-five. This means that at least one in twenty people under forty-five has what doctors sometimes term a 'rheumatic disorder', one in five between forty-five and sixty-four, and two in five over sixty-five.

Second, arthritis is not trivial. If you have it, even mildly, you'll know that it can be very debilitating. The pain is long-term, or

Introduction

what doctors call chronic, and yet often unpredictable. You may not feel too bad one day and then terrible the next. But it's not just physical; it's mentally draining too – and that, while it might not be caused by wider society's indifference to and lack of understanding of arthritis, is not helped by it. That's why this book will look not only at how arthritis affects your body but also at arthritis and the mind. Arthritis and your pain are real, and they are not your fault.

The third myth to debunk is that you 'just live with it'. You don't. Many of the problems that arthritis brings are not caused by the condition itself, but by how other people and society in general react to it. Many of these problems can therefore be solved by you and others.

This is an example of what I mean. A friend of mine cannot use a standard tin-opener. It makes it difficult for him to prepare meals. What's the real problem? His arthritis or the design of the tin-opener? One of these can be changed very easily indeed.

By seeing problems as the result of medical conditions, we tend to assume they can't be solved without 'curing' the condition itself. With a disease in which the cause is unknown, such as arthritis, a 'cure' is not likely in the near future. And even if a cure were found tomorrow it would not undo the joint damage that has already been caused. That requires magic, not medicine.

It is helpful therefore, however severe or mild your arthritis, to see disability as a social problem rather than a medical one. Approaching your life in this way can enable you to start to solve some of the problems that arthritis brings rather than waiting for medical science to do it for you. It's much easier to do this by talking with other people who understand and, of course, other people with arthritis. Again, more about that later.

The fear trap
People with more severe cases of arthritis may become very seriously impaired. They may have visible joint damage and need to use a wheelchair or other mobility aid. This image can be very frightening for someone newly diagnosed with arthritis – they are worried that they will 'end up' like this too – but it is based on a

misunderstanding of the disease itself and of the experience of disability. Most forms of arthritis are milder than this. Even those which are more severe are only so in a minority of cases, and most people with very severe arthritis lead fulfilling and happy lives. I know many who say that the need to develop skills to deal with their impairment (and others' attitudes to it) has made them stronger people. So don't fall into the fear trap. You may be unconvinced by this at the moment – I hope that by the time you've finished this book you won't be.

You can dip into this book as you wish (although I hope you won't want to put it down!) and I hope you will find it useful – but don't forget that arthritis needs to be diagnosed by a doctor. The information and ideas in here should be seen as supplementary to a thorough consultation with your GP or other health professional, and not a substitute for it.

CHAPTER 2

Types of Arthritis

From the cranium in the skull to the phalanges in the feet, there are more than two hundred bones in the body. There are nearly as many types of arthritis and nearly as many words used to describe it. From twinges, aches and pains (or 'the old Arthur') to unpronounceable medical descriptions. Some commonly used expressions are vague and imprecise. The term 'rheumatism' is widely used in general conversation but rarely by doctors. They prefer to talk of rheumatic diseases.

The word 'arthritis' comes from the Latin 'arthro' which means joint and 'itis' which means inflammation (as in, for example, appendicitis). It is an umbrella term for dozens of often very different conditions. Some do not, in fact, feature inflammation but they all involve the joints in some way or another.

The six parts of a joint
A joint is where two bones meet. The typical joint consists of six parts.

★ **Ligaments** are like elastic cords connecting the bones together.
★ **Cartilage** coats the end of each bone, providing a cushion to prevent them rubbing against each other. The gristle you find in meat is actually cartilage.
★ The joint is surrounded by a **synovial sac** full of synovial fluid which lubricates the joint rather like oil (although it is much more effective than the stuff you put in your car engine).
★ The **muscles** are 'elastic' body tissue that enable us to move our joints.

Getting a Grip

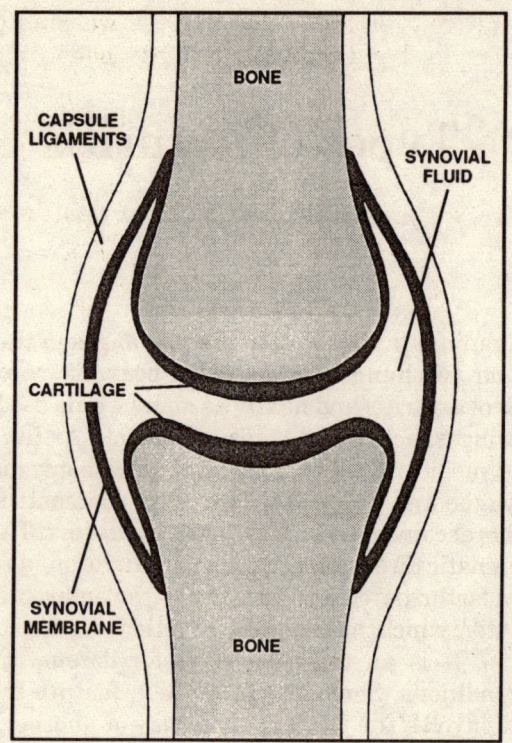

★ **Tendons** connect the muscles to the joint. You can feel two tendons at the back of your knee, one on either side.
★ The movement of the muscles themselves is lubricated by the fluid in the **bursa sac**, which operates in a similar way to the synovial fluid around the joint.

When something goes wrong with one or more of these parts, arthritis can be the result.

The six categories of arthritis

★ Inflammatory – diseases which begin with swelling in the synovial membrane. For example, rheumatoid arthritis.

★ Degenerative – diseases in which the wearing away of the cartilage leaves bone rubbing against bone. For example, osteoarthritis.
★ Periarticular – diseases which occur not in the joint itself but outside it where the tendons and ligaments join the bone. For example, ankylosing spondylitis.
★ Crystals – diseases which result from crystals forming in the joint. For example, gout.
★ Infective – diseases arising from viruses or bacteria in the joint. That is, reactive arthritis.
★ Muscular – diseases of the muscle. These are not strictly speaking forms of arthritis but the symptoms can be similar. For example, fibrositis and certain types of back pain.

The next section looks at some of the most common forms of arthritis. Of course, all diseases are best diagnosed by a doctor, but this is particularly important in the case of arthritis because it can be very difficult to diagnose. The information here should not be used for self-diagnosis. If you think you may have arthritis, make an appointment with your GP.

OSTEOARTHRITIS

Osteoarthritis is the most common form of arthritis. After cardiovascular (heart) disease, it is the major cause of disability in adults. The British League Against Rheumatism, an organisation of health professionals and patients' organisations, estimates that over three million people consult their doctors every year about osteoarthritis. As many as five million people may have the disease.

Osteoarthritis was traditionally regarded as 'wear and tear' arthritis, the inevitable result of ageing. This is not so. The disease is more common in older people because the joint's own repair mechanism deteriorates, but it can affect anyone of any age at any time. It generally comes on relatively slowly. The cartilage becomes worn and roughens and bony lumps form which may make the joint appear knobbly. As the cartilage becomes more worn so the bones begin to rub together. This can be very painful and may cause the joint to change shape. The synovial sac may become inflamed.

The term osteoarthritis is not particularly accurate because, by and large, inflammation is not involved. Osteoarthrosis would probably be more appropriate, but osteoarthritis remains the term used. When doctors talk generally about inflammatory arthritis they do not mean osteoarthritis because joint inflammation is not usually a major feature.

Osteoarthritis most commonly affects the knees, hips, hands, feet and spine. Because there are so many joints in the spine, it is particularly vulnerable. The neck and lower back are most usually affected. Osteoarthritis in the hip and knee may well worsen more quickly than in other joints, some of which may remain stable for years.

Unlike rheumatoid arthritis, osteoarthritis is not a systemic disease affecting the whole body; it tends to affect specific joints – sites of old sports injuries, for example. Affected joints tend to be more painful at the end of the day and after exercise. On the other hand, they will become stiff if left inactive.

Osteoarthritis varies considerably from individual to individual. Some people with mild OA may never realise they actually have it, while for others it is very disabling and may result in the need for surgery. Because the disease is often regarded simply as a sign of ageing, and as its symptoms are so difficult to observe clinically, it can be very hard to get a prompt diagnosis or even a particularly sympathetic response from health professionals. Don't be put off. Your pain is serious and so is osteoarthritis.

RHEUMATOID ARTHRITIS

Rheumatoid arthritis usually begins at a younger age than osteoarthritis, commonly when you are in your thirties. It affects three times as many women as men. About 1% of the population has what rheumatologists call 'definite' rheumatoid arthritis, but many more will have it in a milder form – perhaps as many as one million people in the UK. However, there is some evidence that the incidence and severity of rheumatoid arthritis is decreasing.

Rheumatoid arthritis is the result of the body's immune system going wrong. In autoimmune diseases – lupus is another example (see page 13) – the immune system, which normally protects the body, turns on it and attacks it. Nobody is quite sure what causes this to happen but, as you can imagine, it is a subject of keen interest to researchers. There is more about the immune system on page 53.

When the autoimmune system is working properly, inflammation is a good thing – a sign that the body is successfully repelling invaders. In rheumatoid arthritis it results in inflammation of the synovial membrane and damage to the ligaments, tendons, cartilage, and to the joint and joint sac. The disease usually begins in the hands and feet. They become warm, swollen and tender.

It is not only the joints that are affected in rheumatoid arthritis, it is the whole body. Debilitating tiredness and aching muscles, similar to a severe bout of flu, are very common. The eyes, skin and, in a few cases, other organs, may also be affected. For this reason, rheumatoid arthritis is often referred to as rheumatoid disease.

By contrast with osteoarthritis, rheumatoid arthritis tends to affect the joints in a symmetrical way, that is, both hips or both knees or both feet. Stiffness is most evident in the mornings.

In older people the disease may come on suddenly. In younger people it may take longer – gradually affecting more joints over a period of months – or it may be what doctors call 'palindromic', that is, the arthritis flares up and eases again intermittently before finally setting in. These 'flare-ups' are also common in active rheumatoid arthritis.

Rheumatoid arthritis is usually diagnosed using blood tests as well as clinical examination. There is more about these tests in Chapter 4.

In about one-third of cases, there is a high rate of remission. That is to say the disease is fairly mild and does not leave severe long-term problems. Another third will be moderately affected, and a further third will have what doctors term a more 'aggressive' disease.

BACK PAIN

It costs the NHS an estimated £350 million, British industry getting on for £3 billion in lost production, and the nation nearly sixty million working days a year. It's back pain.

Most people will experience back pain at some point in their lives – it appears to be an occupational hazard of walking upright. Problems are particularly common in the neck (called the cervical region by doctors) and the lower back (called the lumbar region).

The thirty-three bones of the spine can be divided into five groups.

★ The neck region – at the top, seven 'cervical' vertebrae (vertebrae are the disc-shaped bones that you can feel when you run your finger down your spine).
★ Next come twelve 'thoracic' vertebrae, providing the spinal protection for the chest.
★ Then there are the five 'lumbar' vertebrae.
★ Next is the sacrum – five bones usually effectively fused as one.
★ And finally the coccyx – again these four tiny bones are joined as one.

The joints of the spine are not of the synovial type described at the start of this chapter. They need to move far less than say the knee or elbow, and the bones are simply separated by what can best be described as cartilage shock absorbers. However, with many of these bones being so very tiny, and with as many as 150 joints in the spinal region, it is perhaps no wonder that so many people have back problems.

Neck pain
Neck problems may arise from a particular incident such as a whiplash injury (resulting from a sudden thrusting forwards and back of the unsupported head). This often happens in a car accident. Other neck problems develop over a longer period – the result of an awkward sleeping position, poor posture or working position, or a combination of all these and more.

Most neck conditions involve restricted head movement – looking over your shoulder, for example, may be difficult. You may also experience muscle spasms and tender vertebrae.

Lower-back pain
Lower-back pain is perhaps even more difficult for doctors to be precise about. This frustration is one of the reasons they may appear unsympathetic to your problem. Most lumbar pain conditions rejoice in the description 'non-specific back pain'. They can follow heavy physical work or long periods in abnormal postures such as in a car or when gardening.

Osteoarthritis of the spine – called lumbar spondylosis – will have similar symptoms: pain and perhaps some stiffness. It is important to see your GP if you have back pain because prompt treatment can prevent long-term problems. Also, back pain can be a symptom of something potentially more serious, such as ankylosing spondylitis.

ANKYLOSING SPONDYLITIS

This most difficult to pronounce of all the forms of arthritis is actually very aptly named once the words are translated. Ankylosing is Greek for stiffness, while spondylitis means inflammation of the spine. After osteoarthritis and rheumatoid arthritis, it is the third most common rheumatic disorder in the country. There are around 80,000 people in the UK with ankylosing spondylitis.

The disease tends to come on in your late teens or early twenties and particularly affects men. Doctors put the ratio at about five men to one woman, although the patients' organisation, the National Ankylosing Spondylitis Society, puts the figure at nearer two and a half to one.

It usually starts in the lower back: the base of the spine, pelvis and hips. The inflammation results in scar tissue forming between the vertebrae. This tissue may eventually fill the space between the bones and become bone itself. The joint stiffens and becomes immobile. Over the years, the pain and stiffness tend to come and go, often disappearing completely by the time you reach your fifties. The eyes are also affected in one in three cases, becoming bloodshot and painful.

Because of the potential locking of the spine, the importance of early diagnosis is obvious. If it is promptly treated – and the main treatment is exercise – this can be avoided.

GOUT

To get gout, you do not have to be an overweight, port-sodden old gentleman. But it helps. The disease affects men much more than women – the ratio may be as high as twenty to one – and alcohol and weight, while not causing gout, are involved in it.

Gout is actually the result of uric acid crystals in the joints. We all have uric acid in our blood, but usually pass it in our urine. If this does not happen, or if you produce too much in the first place, crystals can grow in the cartilage or joint space.

High levels of uric acid tend to run in families, but no single gene seems to be responsible. In fact, most people with high uric acid levels do not develop gout.

Gout affects the feet, especially the big toe, the ankles, hands and wrists. It can be very painful – although an attack usually lasts only a few days – and can damage the cartilage.

Because it is known specifically what causes gout, it is one of the few forms of arthritis that can be readily cured. Both drugs – usually allopurinal (brand name: Zyloric) – and diet can be used to reduce the amounts of uric acid in the body. Losing weight may also help. If anti-inflammatory drugs are used then aspirin should be avoided as this can increase the level of uric acid. (More about drugs in Chapter 5.)

Although gout is not actually caused by food or drink, certain foods – such as those high in purines – and drinks can make matters worse, and are best monitored closely if you have the disease. These are:

★ foods – game, pâté, offal (liver, sweetbreads and kidney), some

fish (shellfish, fish roe, salmon, herring and whitebait), yeast and its extracts, strawberries, rhubarb, spinach and asparagus
★ drinks – port and carbonated drinks including beer, champagne and sparkling wine

SYSTEMIC LUPUS ERYTHEMATOSUS

Systemic lupus erythematosus, usually called SLE or simply lupus, is still a rare rheumatic disease. The immune system is involved in a similar way to rheumatoid arthritis but, unlike RA, lupus appears to be increasing. Traditional estimates of the prevalence of the disease would put the number of people with SLE in the UK at around 4,000 but this is generally thought to be an underestimate.

The apparent increase in the number of cases may be as much or more the result of improved diagnostic techniques than of any actual increase. In other words, doctors are simply getting better at detecting the disease. They are also getting better at treating it. Lupus can still kill in its most severe forms, but this is becoming much much rarer.

The disease affects eight or nine women to every one man, and is most common among women of child-bearing age. There is some evidence to suggest it might be more common in black people than in white.

It affects not only the joints – although it rarely causes joint damage – but also the tendons and skin and, in some cases, the other organs of the body, notably the kidneys. Inflammation of the body's internal organs can occur occasionally – in the lungs, for example, causing chest pains.

The classic sign of lupus is supposedly a red flushing across the cheeks. This was considered to make the face look rather like a wolf's and gave the disease its name – lupus is Latin for wolf. The name does not seem particularly apt. This flushing appears in fewer than half of lupus cases and you need a vivid imagination to see its resemblance to the features of a wolf. Clearly the name was coined by a doctor rather than a vet.

When the disease flares up, it is not unlike rheumatoid arthritis: the immune system appears to be turning on itself, there is joint and muscle pain, and you feel feverish and fluey. However, it is perhaps easier to see arthritis as a symptom of lupus rather than lupus as a type of arthritis. It can vary greatly from person to person – one of the reasons why it used to be so difficult to diagnose. Like RA, it can also come and go over the years.

Sunlight can trigger a flare-up and will certainly make any skin rashes worse.

If you have SLE and are pregnant, it is particularly important to keep your doctor fully informed as pregnancy may make the disease worse.

REACTIVE ARTHRITIS

Reactive arthritis is inflammation in the joints as a result of an infection elsewhere in the body, for example a viral infection such as a sore throat. There may well be a delay of as much as six weeks between becoming infected and the beginning of the arthritis and, even once the infection is treated, arthritis may still result.

Reactive arthritis is usually relatively short-lived. It generally affects only a few joints, usually one or two larger ones – the knee, elbow or ankle are typical – and rarely affects both of a pair of joints. Sometimes a toe swells up like a sausage and tendons become inflamed, particularly the Achilles tendons and tendons in the wrist.

Types of infection

★ Infections of the bowel with salmonella or a similar germ, resulting in food poisoning. Most of these clear up on their own, but a few may need treatment with antibiotics.

★ Sexually transmitted infections. Most of the sexually transmitted diseases (STDs) can cause arthritis – which you may consider yet another reason, were one needed, for practising safe sex. The commonest STD which can cause a reactive arthritis is a 'non-specific urethritis' caused by the Chlamydia organism. It is passed on during sex and so both partners need to consult a doctor, either your GP or at an STD (or genito-urinary) clinic.

In both types, an off-white discharge from the vagina or penis may well be one of the symptoms of infection. Other symptoms can include a high temperature, ulcers and skin rashes on the soles of the feet and palms.

One particular type of reactive arthritis, where inflammation also occurs in the eye (resulting in conjunctivitis or irisitis), is called Reiter's Disease after the German military doctor who, in the trenches of the First World War, first identified the syndrome.

The arthritis that results from the initial infection involves inflammation in the synovial membrane. It may be more painful in the morning. At first, it will be very active but usually goes into remission after a few months.

Reactive arthritis is twenty times more common in men than women. It is in the same group of diseases within the arthritis 'family' as ankylosing spondylitis and, as with AS, is more common in people with the particular cell group HLA B27. However, as this group makes up more than 10% of the population, there are vastly more HLA B27s without reactive arthritis or ankylosing spondylitis than there are with.

PSORIATIC ARTHRITIS

Psoriasis, from the Greek word for itch, is a fairly common skin disease affecting some 1% of the population. It is not contagious in any way. Skin, usually that of the elbows, knees and scalp, becomes inflamed and red, appearing almost scaly. It is not the result of too much or too little washing. In fact, it has nothing to do with hygiene.

'Normal' skin cells live three to five weeks, working their way to the surface before flaking off unnoticed. Psoriatic cells do all this inside a week, dragging live cells with them to the skin's surface and causing a rash.

In about 5% of cases, arthritis is also present. This suggests perhaps 30,000 people in the UK have psoriatic arthritis. It is a particularly unpredictable form of the disease. Strictly speaking, psoriatic arthritis is a misleading description because it suggests one disease. Psoriasis is actually present in a number of types of arthritis and nobody really understands the link between them. What they have in common is inflammation and a tendency to wax and wane over time.

Psoriasis may appear by pure coincidence in rheumatoid arthritis, or it may signify not RA but psoriatic arthropathy. This appears similar to RA but particularly causes painful swollen fingertips and tends to affect fewer joints. Psoriasis can also appear alongside ankylosing spondylitis.

Psoriatic arthritis mutilans is the particularly severe form of the disease that often requires hospital treatment. Television dramatist Dennis Potter drew on his own personal experience of this condition in his acclaimed BBC series *The Singing Detective*.

ARTHRITIS IN CHILDREN

Although this is a self-help book for adults, it is worth saying a few words about arthritis in children, if only to disprove one of the most common myths about the disease. Moreover, some readers may recognise some of these symptoms from their childhoods.

There are 15,000 under-sixteens with arthritis in this country, the majority of them girls. Doctors divide so-called Juvenile Chronic Arthritis (or JCA) into three different types.

★ Systemic – affects the whole body and usually begins in very young children. The child may be feverish and have body rashes. Body temperature fluctuates and joints are painful. It is sometimes called Still's Disease after the doctor who first identified it.

★ Poly-articular – affects the joints specifically rather than the whole body, although the child may feel generally unwell. It is usually symmetrical involving many (poly meaning many) large joints.

★ Pauci-articular – affects fewer joints, four or less, usually beginning in just one. Eye problems may occur, so regular eye-tests are essential, but generally there is little effect on the child's general health.

Not all children with arthritis have one of the above. Some have juvenile versions of ankylosing spondylitis, rheumatoid arthritis or psoriatic arthritis.

Although symptoms and treatment are similar for children and adults, the problems children face as a result can of course be very different. Many children do not go on to experience arthritis in their adult lives, but some do. Joints may be damaged and growth affected.

The voluntary organisation Arthritis Care has a special section, 'Young Arthritis Care', which can help young people with arthritis and their parents. It runs courses and produces books and magazines.

MUSCULAR MANIFESTATIONS

As we said above, muscular problems, being outside the joints, are not strictly types of arthritis, and some doctors working in rheumatology are very sceptical about them. They are dubious about both the symptoms (some say they are 'all in the mind') and their classification in 'their' field. Not very helpful for those with the conditions!

Fibrositis is probably quite common among the over fifties, affecting perhaps 10,000 people. It is caused by the muscles never really relaxing. They remain tense all day and often even all night, putting strain on the ligaments. It is painful and sleep may be disturbed. Appropriate exercise and relaxation can help.

Polymyalgia Rheumatica is rarer. The cause is unknown but it results in tenderness in the hips, neck and shoulders. It is particularly painful in the morning and worsens again later in the day. You can also feel tired and depressed and lose some weight. It may be treated successfully with steroids.

Fibromyalgia is the real focus of controversy among medics. People experience widespread, ill-defined pain and sleep is disturbed. Again depression and other symptoms that may be psychological rather than physical are present, and this is the problem. There is no doubt that many lives are severely affected by this condition, but doctors remain divided on whether there are genuine physical symptoms that require treatment. Some argue that it is the underlying social and psychological causes that need attention.

OSTEOPOROSIS

Whereas arthritis is strictly speaking a disease of the joints, osteoporosis is a disease of the bones. Like the rest of your body, bones are living tissue – cells are constantly being replaced. Although this does slow as we get older – maximum bone strength occurs between thirty and forty years old – if it stops happening at a sufficient rate, the bones can become thinner and more brittle. This is osteoporosis. It can cause pain in the bones, particularly the spine and hips, and lead to fractures.

Osteoporosis is more common in older people, particularly post-menopausal women. In this age group, it affects one in four women and one in forty men. It is more common in white-skinned people and those who are lightly built.

You are at increased risk of osteoporosis if:

★ your menopause comes early
★ a close relative has the disease
★ you have been using oral steroids or antacids – both of which are used in treating arthritis – for a long time (injected steroids appear to be less of a problem)
★ your calcium and vitamin D intakes have been low, particularly as a child
★ you do not or are unable to take sufficient exercise
★ you have had certain other diseases of the liver, thyroid or lungs

Types of Arthritis

These risks are exacerbated by cigarette smoking and high levels of alcohol consumption.

People with osteoarthritis may, because the bone mass tends to increase in osteoarthritis, be at less of a risk of osteoporosis. As the above list demonstrates, there are a number of other factors involved. However, the risk of osteoporosis is higher in people with rheumatoid arthritis because oral steroids can deplete the calcium in the bones.

The female hormone oestrogen reduces the body's ability to dissolve bone and stimulates the body's production of vitamin D and calcitonin, which also helps maintain bones. When the production of oestrogen stops with the menopause, the risk of osteoporosis is clearly increased. An early sign of osteoporosis may be reduced height after the menopause.

If you are a woman at risk of osteoporosis, talk to your doctor about Hormone Replacement Therapy (HRT). This involves taking oestrogen by mouth, skin patch or by means of a small implant beneath the skin. Ideally you should discuss this before your menopause begins, although the treatment can be started ten to fifteen years after menstruation ends. As with all treatments there are risks to consider. Although some people sleep better and have more energy as a result, others feel 'unnatural'. There is an increased risk of breast cancer. There is also an increased risk of cancer of the uterus, but this may be offset by taking the other female hormone progesterone with the oestrogen. Another type of treatment, such as calcitonin or ethidronate drugs, may help if HRT is unsuitable (for example, if you are a man!).

Although some specific exercises can help once your bone mass is reduced, osteoporosis is best prevented at an earlier stage by a healthy diet, particularly in childhood, and regular weight-bearing exercise, especially in your middle years and upwards. Weight-bearing exercise is that where the bones must support your weight. They respond to this demand by increasing the calcium content and thus their strength. Swimming, for example, is not a weight-bearing exercise. Walking is. If you can, just half a mile a day helps.

Because these simple preventative strategies can be successful, it is important that people with arthritis, particularly younger women with RA, are aware of the risks of osteoporosis. Exercise is discussed in more detail in Chapter 9, and diet in Chapter 7.

SJOGREN'S SYNDROME

This syndrome, identified by Swedish physician Henrik Sjogren in 1933, affects half a million people in the UK, primarily women. Its distinctive features are dry eyes and a dry mouth. It may affect these parts of the face alone but more commonly comes in tandem with arthritis – either rheumatoid arthritis, systemic lupus erythematosus, or a similar disease.

Like RA and lupus, Sjogren's syndrome is an autoimmune disease in which the immune system turns in on itself. In this case it destroys the mucus-producing glands (called the exocrine glands). Other symptoms may include a general flu-like feeling, as in other autoimmune diseases, and skin rashes. In rare cases the kidneys and liver may become involved.

As yet, doctors are unable to restore glandular secretions, but artificial tears and saliva are available. Anti-inflammatories and other drugs commonly used in the treatment of arthritis are also employed.

WORK-RELATED ARTHRITIS

Is work bad for you?
Day-to-day activity has always been a major factor in the development of arthritis and related conditions. Think of 'tennis elbow' (where the point at which the tendon joins the bone is damaged) or 'housemaid's knee' (where a bursa becomes damaged and swollen). The mind boggles at the occupation of someone with the condition in which a swollen tendon in the finger can become stuck in a flexed position. It's called 'trigger finger'.

You may think the notion of repetitive strain injuries, the expression often used today for work-related forms of arthritis, is a new one. It's not. In the fifties it was reported that mining caused arthritis in the knees and spine. In the sixties, French farmers were shown to be five times as likely to develop osteo-arthritis as other workers. As long ago as 1964, the Japanese were already talking about what they called occupational disorders and trying to limit the number of keystrokes performed by typists, telephonists and similar workers. What is new is that work-related arthritis of the repetitive strain injury type is now in the headlines. And it's not surprising.

Today's technology is tomorrow museum's piece. Working conditions are changing more rapidly now than at any time since the industrial revolution. Yet repetitive injuries, by their very nature, take time to become apparent. Who knows what occupational time-bomb we might be building our economy on? The snowballing of repetitive strain injury cases – trades unions have dozens and dozens awaiting settlement; employers are often happy to settle out of court – is a hint of what might be there.

From shooting down a space invader to preparing the quarterly accounts; from typing a letter to talking to Tokyo, computers can do it. As computer technology gets faster and faster and it becomes possible to do more and more on it, any dangers arising from repetitive actions at keyboards must increase.

When there's a personal computer on every desk, it's not just secretaries who need nimble fingers on the keyboard. Microsoft, probably the world's leading computer software company, now includes cigarette-style health warnings on its keyboards. In the American courts, computer giant IBM is facing accusations that it has known about the dangers of using a conventional keyboard for years but didn't tell its customers, only its staff. The computer industry is perhaps understandably reluctant to accept some of the problems its product brings. Doctors have no excuse.

Repetitive strain injuries (RSI), or work-related upper-limb disorders (WRULD) as they are sometimes known, are the result of a combination of factors, not simply the use of a keyboard – but it all boils down to the fact that continual repetition of the same tiny movement time and again is potentially dangerous.

There are two main causes of RSI:

★ Static posture – standing or sitting in the same position for hours contracts the same muscles and squeezes the same nerves and blood vessels. Oxygen has trouble circulating.
★ Repetition – using the same muscles to do the same thing time and again.

The effect of these will vary from individual to individual and from workplace to workplace. Static posture and repetition along with the following could result in RSI:

★ Individual factors – for example, bad posture and difficulties handling stress.
★ Environmental factors – for example, badly designed or unreliable work-stations and stressful working environments. (It is the stress of continual deadlines that probably explains why journalists seem so susceptible to RSI.) A stressful working environment will exaggerate tensions in the muscles.

These are the medical names of the most common forms of repetitive strain injury. They are all of the periarticular type: that is, outside the joint.

★ Tenosyvitis – inflammation of the synovial sheath around the tendons which prevents it releasing enough synovial fluid for the tendon to move smoothly.
★ Tendinitis – inflammation of the tendons themselves.
★ Carpal Tunnel Syndrome – inflammation presses on the nerve which passes through the so-called carpal tunnel which runs down the arm to the hand. Pins and needles and numbness accompany pain.
★ Peritendinitis – inflammation around the point where the tendon joins the muscle.
★ Epicondylitis – the medical term for 'tennis elbow'. Inflammation where the muscle joins the bone.

OTHER TYPES OF ARTHRITIS

There are many other types of arthritis. Most are related to one or other of the diseases already described. They can, however, bring their own particular difficulties. There is not space here to go into detail, but a full list of support organisations for the many varieties of arthritis appears in Chapter 13.

IS ARTHRITIS HEREDITARY?

Certain types of arthritis appear to run in families, but that knowledge is not necessarily as helpful as you might imagine. Quite how remains a mystery.

The question is often asked, because people wonder if they will get arthritis if a parent had it or if they will pass their own arthritis on to their children. This cannot be precisely answered. In studies of identical twins, where both have exactly the same genes, it is unusual for both to develop arthritis. This suggests there must be more to it than heredity alone.

The Arthritis and Rheumatism Council, the UK's major arthritis research organisation, conclude in their booklet that: 'The chances of an affected parent directly handing on the disease to his or her children are very small indeed.'

There is no arthritis gene passing from generation to generation although, on the face of it, a particular white blood cell molecule called HLA B27 should be a candidate. It is present in over 90% of people with ankylosing spondylitis and also very commonly found in people with reactive arthritis and psoriatic arthritis. However, HLA B27 is not rare – a tenth of the population has it – and probably 98% of people with HLA B27 never develop arthritis.

Similarly, systemic lupus erethymatosus is associated with an excess in the blood of what are called autoantibodies. Rheumatoid arthritis is associated with both HLA and autoantibodies.

People with these patterns in their own blood could be said to have a 'genetic predisposition' to the disease, but the disease itself is triggered by an external factor. This is perhaps easiest to see in the case of reactive arthritis. The disease itself is discussed in more detail above, but suffice to say that one type of reactive arthritis results from a sexually transmitted infection. A study of soldiers in the seventies found that HLA B27 was no more common among those with the sexually transmitted infection than among those without. However, it was present in the vast majority of those with the infection who then went on to develop arthritis. In other words, people with HLA B27 were no more likely to get the infection than anyone else but, if they did get it, it was far more likely to trigger arthritis.

Dr Derek Brewerton, in his book *All About Arthritis*, an investigative history of arthritis research, suggests something similar happens with ankylosing spondylitis, psoriatic arthritis and rheumatoid arthritis. He says that it is 'host factors' – that is, things to do with the individual, including heredity, age, sex, reactions to stress, nutrition and so on – that will determine how a disease progresses, whether it remains a mild inflammation or develops into more severe arthritis – but these things will not actually cause it.

To summarise, arthritis is not inherited, although a 'genetic disposition' to it may be. The arthritis is probably triggered by something outside the individual. However, this is not the same for each person. (If arthritis *is* caused by a specific germ, as nineteenth-century physicians believed, it has eluded detection for a century; this seems unlikely.)

Rheumatoid factor

In 1937 an unusual protein was discovered in the blood of people with rheumatoid arthritis. The scientist involved, Erik Waaler from Norway, unsure of what he had discovered, called it rheumatoid factor. At least 70% of people with rheumatoid arthritis have it in their blood, but whether it is a cause or an effect of the disease is unknown. There is some evidence that those with a particularly high rheumatoid factor develop a more severe disease.

However, rheumatoid factor is found in the blood of 5% of the population – in other words, over three-quarters of people with rheumatoid factor do not have arthritis.

CHAPTER 3

How Do You Feel?

Phew, that's the medical stuff over with. But perhaps the next bit is even harder because it's about you.

Obviously it's important to get a medical diagnosis for what you're feeling from a doctor. So much the better if they can tell you which type of arthritis you have got. The many forms of the disease are very different. We feel better once our condition has a name, once the suggestions that we have all heard of how it's 'all in the mind' can be rebutted. So, you have arthritis, what next? Diagnosis is not the end of it, not even the beginning of the end. This is a long-term condition, after all. The important thing is that you are now in a position to begin to take control.

It may be tempting to try to find out more and more medical information about your disease, to read every book and become an amateur rheumatologist: the Miss Marple of musculo-skeletal disorders. Equally, you might feel like never thinking about it again and just getting on with your life. Since being diagnosed, most of you have quite possibly felt like doing both. However, neither is any good in the long-term because they both rely on a blind faith, a triumph of hope over experience.

You can read every book ever written on the subject, talk to every rheumatologist – and obviously there is value in doing this – but you won't find the hidden treasure, the magic solution that will turn everything back to 'normal'. The cure. Scientists have been looking for it for years – they still are – but even if they find it, who says it is going to help you? Things certainly won't go back to being the way they were.

Thinking about how we feel is an important starting point for dealing with any change. In the case of a medical condition which may well last a long time and could affect many aspects of our life, it is essential.

In this chapter we meet three people with different types of arthritis and learn about how the disease affects their lives, what's happened to them and how they feel about it. They all have more significant arthritis, but they're not particularly exceptional or unusual people. They all have different forms of the disease and are of different ages. Perhaps between them they've had more than their fair share of unsympathetic and unhelpful professionals, but the thing they all have in common is that, despite this, they have forged their own way. By accepting their disease they have found their own ways to live with it. Between them Joy, Chris and Margaret raise most of the topics covered in this book, so if you're newly diagnosed and not always sure what they're talking about, don't worry – you'll find it all in a later chapter (or try the index).

JOY'S STORY

Joy Scarlett is fifty-five and has osteoarthritis.

'I got arthritis in 1972 as the result of a road traffic accident, a car crash. I suffered disc compression in the spine and my walking was affected. However, they put my subsequent problems down to stress after the accident.

'I was working as a nurse then, on a children's fracture ward, but even so it seemed like the end of the world. It's the not knowing. If you don't know what's happening you can't come to terms with it and move forward.

'While I was still off sick after the accident, I was sent to a rehabilitation unit where the doctor said there was more wrong than I'd been told. I've a lot to thank him for. He sent me to a rheumatology unit. All in all, it took eighteen months before arthritis was diagnosed.

'I was put on ibuprofen (an anti-inflammatory drug) and I was on it for fifteen years. Eventually I said to my doctor that I was worried my stomach would be damaged. She said, "If your stomach was going to go it would have done so years ago." Then eighteen months ago I got a peptic ulcer. I went back to the doctor and challenged her. She said, "What was the point of me alarming you?" '

Ulcers are a not uncommon side-effect from anti-inflammatory drugs. 'If anything the ulcer has been worse than the arthritis. It was the ulcer that caused my retirement from work. I'd moved from nursing to the Department of Employment and I'd been there for fifteen years. I'd never had a day off with the arthritis. They used the opportunity provided by my being off with the ulcer to get rid of me.' Ironically, Joy was an assistant disability employment adviser, helping other people with disabilities to get back into work. Now she's applying for part-time jobs. She's also very active in the voluntary organisation Arthritis Care. What helps with her arthritis?

'Well, I'm only on painkillers now because of the ulcer. The TENS machine [see page 71] is extremely good, but because I have spinal arthritis I can't bend my body enough to actually attach it to the affected parts – the daft thing is of course that it's particularly difficult on the days I really need it.

'I also use aromatherapy. I found it in a magazine and sent for the oils. My sister, who is a nurse, makes them up for me and other people with arthritis. I rub them into my skin two or three times a day. It doesn't last long, but it's very soothing and smells lovely. Of course it's not cheap but disabilities aren't cheap. Many people don't realise this.

'I used to do hydrotherapy every week for about twenty minutes. A senior physiotherapist helped with the exercises. It's amazing how much exercise you can do in that lovely warm water that you can't do on land. The problem is that, on the NHS, it's not available everywhere and if it is it's usually only for a short time. Our Arthritis Care group hired the hydro pool so we could all go regularly – we took thirty to forty people – but then the hospital closed it because it was too expensive. Now it's sitting there doing nothing. The nearest one is eighteen miles away. I miss that – I've got slowly stiffer.

'Exercise is vitally important, but so is rest. The difficult bit is the balance. Too much rest and you get stiff; too much exercise and you're in pain. I relax in my garden. If I'm uptight I just disappear out there. I don't do much – just a bit of dead-heading or something – but afterwards I'm a different person.

'I do my stretching exercises anywhere – watching TV, even in traffic jams – you get some funny looks!

'I've discovered that citric acid doesn't seem to agree with me, so I try to keep that out of my diet. I don't know if it specifically affects my arthritis but I certainly feel better for avoiding it.

'I'd have to say that arthritis has affected my personal relationships. I haven't had a close relationship for some time. There's a fear of the unknown – walking funnily as I do.

'When I first had it, it was difficult for everybody. People wanted to do too much. Now family and friends know there isn't anything I can't do – it just takes time. Initially I was terribly ungracious, but the truth is: if you don't know how to handle your arthritis, how can you expect other people to know how to handle it?

'I have been very proud over the years. I didn't want to appear different. Now it doesn't bother me. Sometimes I used a wheelchair at work. It made me self-sufficient. Without it, I wouldn't have done half of what I did, I wouldn't have been able to carry anything – and I still had enough energy left when I got home to do my housework and voluntary work.

'Colleagues found it hard to come to terms with. They see you walking one day and using a wheelchair the next. I've stopped trying to justify it. If people can't accept me as I am, forget it.

'A lot of problems are caused by other people's attitudes. I don't want sympathy and I don't want to be patronised. I could have knocked the block off one rheumatologist. Now I'm better able to talk to doctors. I usually know more about it than they do.

'Arthritis has made me a much better person. I can now appreciate others' problems much more than I could before – even though I used to think that I could. I'm sorry I had to have it, but it has enhanced my life – I have much more empathy.'

CHRIS'S STORY

Chris Hogg is thirty-nine. His tendinitis is the result of a repetitive strain injury at work.

'I began in the print trade twenty-two years ago as an apprentice typesetter. I worked in nine or ten places, moving around, moving up. I finished up in London doing magazine work – advertisement setting. It's high-pressure work. They have a lot of money to chuck about and they want what they want when they want it. I was doing between ten and sixteen hours a day, five nights a week, and without a break, for about a year.

'Previously, in the mid-eighties when I'd been doing nights, I'd had tendinitis, but that went away after six months, when I stopped doing nights. Obviously, tiredness in a high-pressure environment was the trigger for me.

'Anyway, it started to happen again. It was the middle of the recession. There were pay cuts. The employers really took advantage, because for every job in the building there were 150 people keen to take your place. The trade union, the NGA, had been kicked into touch. Every night someone would come in and say such and such a place had shut.

'I had pain in the top of my shoulder as I'd had before. I daren't go sick because they were already making people redundant at our place. I just slapped on cream and heat treatments all day. It got worse and worse. I was doing everything with my right arm and then I got it in there as well. I was terrified and went sick. This was late 1990.

'I went back just before Christmas, but I didn't last a week. I had to go home one night. I was nearly in tears – everyone is looking at you, thinking you're skiving, putting it on, they know you don't like nights. I was off sick for three months. People were being made redundant and one Saturday morning my letter came.

'Meanwhile, my GP had diagnosed tendinitis fairly early on, but I had to wait ten weeks for physio in which time it got worse. Once I started it took me six to twelve months to realise that NHS physios don't have a clue about this condition. They just wheeled me round, trying me on everything!

'One of them – the third physio I saw – was from Zimbabwe and she introduced me to ANT stretches – adverse neural tension – controlled stretches of the tendon, which are probably the only effective form of treatment for RSI. Unfortunately she left after three weeks.

'I had to start again. The others tried to do the stretches when I told them about them but they were clueless. All my rheumatologist could offer was cortisone injections. I had two in the same site and they didn't work. When he wanted to give me a third I said no.

'The first two times I'd seen him privately and he was as nice as ninepence – obsequious, even. The third time was on the NHS and he treated me like dirt. Didn't look at me the entire time, just at his notes. I don't even know if they were my notes or his next private patient. When I said no to the injection, he just closed the file and that was it.

'The next consultant – private again – referred me to a private physio, but again there was no improvement and the same high staff turnover. I was paying £30 a go to bring them up to speed! I've seen eleven physios altogether now, and only the third one and the last one knew what they were doing. Now I use the exercises and stretches the last one showed me in my maintenance programme and it really does work.

'All this time I'm on Social Security benefits. I felt a completely useless burden – it stops your life, not just your work.

'It was then I discovered computer-based voice-recognition technology. Not that the Disability Employment Adviser at the local Job Centre told me about it. They suggested I read gas meters as it was a walking job that didn't need my hands!'

As a person whose disability affected his ability to work, Chris was entitled to financial help for specialist equipment from the Department of Employment. 'The technology wasn't as advanced as it is now, and I had to do a lot of work to put together a package that would enable me to do the sort of design and typesetting work that I do. Still the authorities weren't very helpful because it was a one-off solution and they didn't understand it.

'Unfortunately you can't have the equipment before you get a job, so you have to persuade employers that it will work – you can't just show them.'

Chris got a print production job with the charity Arthritis Care in spring 1994. 'I'm really glad it was Arthritis Care that offered me a job because a commercial employer wouldn't have waited the time that Arthritis Care waited for the Department of Employment to provide the equipment. It took over six months, and they kept sending the wrong stuff.

'The thing about RSI is that the people who don't care don't get it – the skivers – which shows that stress is a big factor. If you feel you're getting it, I'd go sick before it gets critical and you lose your job. Find a physio who can show you some ANT stretches.

'It's humbling and humiliating not being able to do the things that guys do. I couldn't play with my kids, cut up my food or dry myself after a shower. Sexual foreplay (or afterplay!) is impossible because your hands hurt so much.

'It was excruciating. For example, watching my wife go round a supermarket, load all the shopping, unload it on to the check-out and pack it all at the end. And me just standing there. You think everyone's thinking, "Look at that lazy sod. Doing nothing."

'These experiences have stopped me doing what everybody does naturally – that is, judging by appearances. It's forced me to be resourceful and has proved the strength of my marriage. I'm glad I work for Arthritis Care now and that I'm out of the cut-throat rat race I was in before. A physical or mental problem of some kind was inevitable at the pressure and pace we were working.'

For me, Chris is proof of the importance of talking to others in a similar position to you rather than avoiding them. I also have a repetitive strain injury. If it weren't for Chris I may have had the same difficult journey as he endured before I discovered voice-recognition computer technology – the exact technology I'm using to write this book.

MARGARET'S STORY

Margaret Stephens is forty-seven and has rheumatoid arthritis. Margaret used to work for a major publishing house. Now she runs her own magazine production business from home.

'I went to the doctor when I was just eighteen with a puffy knee. It was diagnosed as fluid on the knee. Then I went to teacher training college in Weymouth. On the back of my father's scooter going to the station I noticed that all my elbows had puffed up too. Within two weeks of arriving in college it was obvious all was not well. I had flaming hot joints.'

But no sooner had Margaret got a diagnosis of rheumatoid arthritis than the flare died down.

'That became the story of my life until 1971. Whenever there was upheaval in my life, it came back. I realised there was a pattern. It would always come back in the autumn. I'd get very tense. I was quite frightened as a person anyway at that time – quite scared of life. I was on indomethacin (an anti-inflammatory drug) every September for about four years.

'In 1969 I went to Australia for two years, had another flare-up during their winter and was on indomethacin again. The problem with this drug was that it made me nauseous and tired all the time. At that time as a young woman this probably had more effect on my life than the arthritis.

'When I returned to England in 1971 – again another upheaval – it came back but this time it didn't go away. The penny dropped very slowly over a couple of years that it wasn't going away this time. It was a cause of great depression and anxiety but very internalised. I was back at teacher training in London. The key thing at that time for a woman of twenty-three, the greatest stress, was trying to hide it. There was a shamefulness attached to it. The desire to be attractive and normal is so strong, very strong.

'Now back in 1966 I had been hospitalised by that first flare, but I didn't see another hospital consultant until 1973 – and even then I had to push for it. I said to my GP should I go to hospital and he said, "No, no, no." A friend's boyfriend, who was a dentist, said if he had what I had, he'd insist. So I did.

'By the time I got to hospital I was not in good shape. Now I make sure I have a peer relationship with any doctor – they are no better than you are. You will get nervous so write things down. One consultant told me, "We don't like lists." I thought, "Tough luck." They think it reduces their control. But don't be too bolshy – your goal is to get the best possible treatment and you won't get this if you alienate your doctor. They're not professional enough to get over the personality thing.'

Margaret's experience demonstrates that you cannot rely on doctors to tell you everything.

'A friend's father told me that you could take indomethacin as a suppository. I put this to my doctor. "Oh yes, you can," they said. "Would you like to try it?" I did. No side-effects except a little wooziness when you're going to bed, which is fine. I'd put up with those terrible side-effects for nine years! The French take a lot of drugs "par anum" because then they largely avoid the stomach.

'A similar thing happened when I went to see the doctor at age forty-three – menopause approaching. I was already thin-boned and was on steroids. I was a classic high risk for osteoporosis, but nobody mentioned hormone replacement therapy. I'd heard you needed to start before the menopause. I said to the doctor, "I think I should do this," and he said, "I suppose you should really." '

While doctors may not tell you everything, others may be keener to share their 'wisdom'. 'I'd heard that dairy products were bad for your arthritis so I didn't eat any for fifteen years, which is absolutely ridiculous. Now I find a low-fat diet has a small but significant benefit for me. I focus on what I can eat – positive – not what I can't eat. But don't be obsessive. Don't screw yourself up emotionally and socially about it.'

What about relationships?

'You often need all your energy to hold yourself together and a routine to suit it. A relationship, someone coming in from the outside, can really rock the boat. Life with arthritis is about management, and in a relationship you have something else to manage. There are fabulous people who are mature and will cope, but it is difficult to go out with someone with a disability. On the other hand, if someone wants you that's their choice. You don't take on responsibility for their problem with your problem.

'If you have a physical disability you do plummet in the attraction shakes. I'd one false hip before I'd told any man about my arthritis, although people must have known.

'Not being married is devastating for many of my single able-bodied friends. For me it's not such a problem. I know how to cope living on my own and being on my own because I've had to come to terms with myself and living within myself.'

AND HOW ABOUT YOU?

How long have you had arthritis? How much time passed between your first symptoms and your diagnosis? Which of these best describes your reaction when you were first diagnosed?

★ Disbelief: 'This doctor doesn't know what he's talking about.' 'I'm not old enough for arthritis.' 'I want a second opinion!'
★ Fear: 'I can't cope with pain.' 'I'll become really ugly.' 'I'll finish up in a wheelchair.'
★ Anger: 'Why me?' 'This is typical of my luck.'
★ Uncertainty: 'What's going to become of me?' 'I'm up and down like a yo-yo – I never know how I'm going to feel.'

You've probably felt all these at some time or other. You may feel some of them now. There's nothing wrong with it. You shouldn't blame yourself for feeling angry or showing your fears. These are understandable reactions. What we need to do is to try to move away from being reactive towards being proactive. In other words, we need to begin to do things rather than simply respond to things that happen to us. The stories of Joy, Chris and Margaret show that it can be difficult, but that, over time, it can be done.

This may involve mourning for what we have lost. Look at the list of emotions again – disbelief, anger, uncertainty, fear – they also all describe how we feel when a relationship ends or someone close to us dies. We feel bereaved. It is necessary for us to recognise the loss of our former, arthritis-free self. Recognise how

How Do You Feel?

you are feeling, accept it, and then move on. This is easier said than done, of course. Sometimes it's very hard to move on. Hopefully this book will provide you with some ways of doing this.

At this stage it might be helpful to stop and think for a few moments about how your feelings have changed towards your arthritis. Try to list the different feelings – they may be some of the ones we have mentioned already or there might be others – and next to each try to say what caused it to change.

Have you been getting more positive or more negative? Probably it has been a bit up and down. Whatever has happened, you are sure to find that there has been some change one way or the other. There will be more than one emotion on your list; your feelings will not have stayed the same.

This shows that our feelings can and will change. If this is so, it makes sense to try to change them to suit us and our well-being.

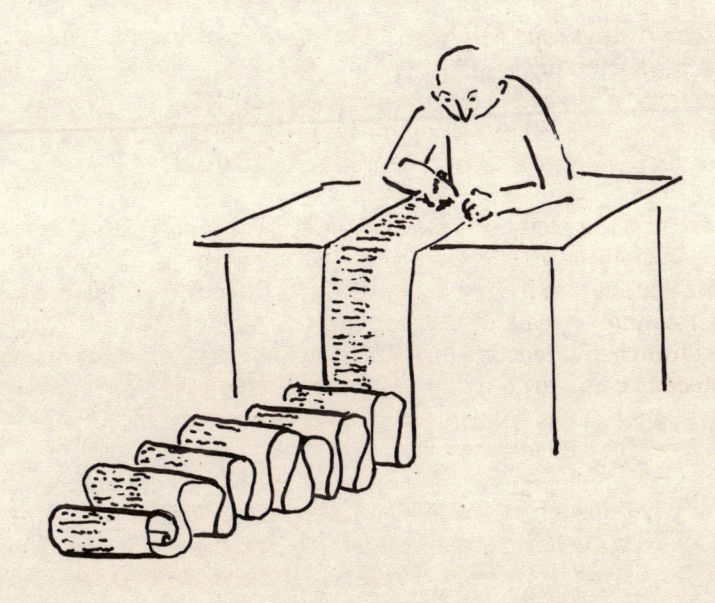

Before leaving this chapter take a sheet of paper (you may need several!) and divide it in half vertically. Down one side make a list of all the problems that your arthritis causes for you – at home, at work, with family and friends, with hobbies, with leisure activities and so on. List as many as you can. Then in the second column, next to each problem, write a solution. It may need something to change in you or other people or even in the environment. It may require something drastic. In some cases you may not be able to think of any solution that doesn't sound fantastical. Write it down anyway. You may not think of a solution for all or even most of your problems. It doesn't matter.

Take some time. When you have given it a good go, put your list to one side and don't return to it until you've finished with this book. That's it for negative thoughts – for the time being at least!

CHAPTER 4

Arthritis and the Health Professionals

You are the most important person in the management of your arthritis. Only you know how you feel. Only you know what your difficulties are and what you actually want help with. However, there are a whole range of others it is sensible to involve, beginning with health professionals.

The National Health Service comes in for a lot of stick these days. It probably isn't as good as it was, but considering that we spend proportionately less public money on it than the US, Canada and most of our European partners, it is still very good indeed and the people who work in it are highly trained and committed.

GENERAL PRACTITIONERS (GP)

Everybody has the right to be registered with a GP, who should be your first port of call for any illness.

It has been estimated that as many as one in four GP appointments concern arthritis. Moreover, a survey by the charity Arthritis Care found that over three-quarters of their members had seen their GP about their arthritis in the previous year. A good relationship with your GP is therefore very important – you could well see a lot of each other.

If you are unable to register with the local GP of your choice – they may already have too many patients, for example – contact your local Family Health Services Authority who can provide you with a full list of general practices in your area.

When you register with a new GP, you should, under the Patients' Charter, be offered an introductory health check. This may well be repeated annually for older patients. When you register, ask for information about the services your practice offers and whether it has its own practice charter. This will outline what you can expect from the practice: opening times, facilities for disabled people and children, arrangements for tests and repeat prescriptions and so on.

If you want to be sure that your GP understands arthritis you could try to track down one of the 300 who are members of the Primary Care Rheumatology Society (PCR), an organisation for GPs with a special interest in arthritis. Ask your GP whether they are a member.

The doctor's ideal approach to any disease is diagnosis followed by treatment. In many cases and particularly with arthritis, this is not possible. Time is an important factor in diagnosis, but your symptoms – pain, swelling, fatigue – need treating immediately. If your doctor sends you away with a prescription but without telling you what the problem is, it doesn't mean he or she doesn't care, simply that he or she doesn't know.

Arthritis is difficult to diagnose, but a good GP should discuss your symptoms with you even if an immediate diagnosis is not possible.

In many cases, to assist in the diagnosis the GP may refer you for blood tests or an X-Ray. In many larger practices these may be done on the premises by a practice nurse. Do not read too much into this – they are as often to rule out certain conditions as to confirm them. The blood tests used in rheumatology are covered below.

At the same time or subsequently, the GP may also refer you on to a specialist, probably a consultant rheumatologist. This does not necessarily mean your problem is too serious for the GP or that they don't know what it is. The specialist is simply that – a specialist, armed with greater knowledge of one particular area of medicine and with a larger battery of diagnostic techniques.

You do not have to see a consultant. Many people manage their arthritis very successfully under the treatment of their GP alone.

However, if you would like to see one, ask your GP. No reasonable request for a referral should be refused.

The Patients' Charter says you have the right to 'be referred to a consultant acceptable to you, when your GP thinks it is necessary, and to be referred for a second opinion if you and your GP agree this is desirable'. In theory this means you should be able to see the consultant you want – and if you do know who you want to see, ask by name – but in practice, although the right might be there, the money might not. This right may be easier to exercise if your GP's practice is a fund-holding one managing its own budget.

A fund-holder can theoretically refer you to any hospital consultant prepared to see you anywhere in the country. Many, however, enter into their own treatment contracts with particular hospitals. They may need persuading to refer outside of these.

Non-fundholding GPs are restricted by the contracts agreed with hospitals and their district health authority. The authority can permit an extra contractual referral to someone else, but there is little money for this.

After referral to a consultant, nine out of ten patients should be seen within thirteen weeks, according to the Charter. Across the country, joint pain is the single biggest reason for a doctor to make a referral to an out-patients' clinic, so it's far from unusual. If you want to be referred, ask.

HOSPITAL CONSULTANTS

Consultants are experts in one particular area of medicine. Those who specialise in arthritis and rheumatic diseases are called rheumatologists. When you are referred you should receive a letter from the relevant hospital asking you to attend an out-patients appointment. If you cannot keep this it is vital that you inform them, otherwise you will lose your place in the queue and deprive someone else of an appointment.

The Royal College of Physicians estimates that there should be one rheumatologist for every 150,000 population. At the turn of the decade, the NHS was the equivalent of ninety-nine full-time consultants short. A study by the Arthritis and Rheumatism Council in 1993 found that Portugal and Eire were the only European countries with a lower rate of rheumatologists per head of population than the UK. The differences are striking. Denmark has 22·4 rheumatologists per 100,000 people; the UK has 3·8. For this reason it can take a long time and possibly a long journey to see a rheumatologist. In general, Northern Ireland, Scotland and Wales tend to be less well-served than England.

The consultant or a member of his or her team may supervise your treatment themselves, refer you back to your GP or refer you on to another health or community professional. In cases of more severe arthritis you may be referred to an orthopaedic surgeon who specialises in joint replacement and other surgery (see below).

Blood tests
'Let's just do a few tests . . .' Sooner or later someone will say this to you. It may be your GP, it may be your consultant. They will then begin talking gobbledegook, uttering meaningless strings of initials and practising tongue-twisters. Don't worry. Neither of you have lost your sanity. Your doctor is simply telling you what tests you are being sent for.

It often seems that the language of medicine has been deliberately created to be as confusing as possible. Medical tests are a prime example – not one seems to have a name that indicates its purpose to the humble patient.

Tests are used in four ways: to assist in diagnosis; to assess a disease's severity; to assess the effects of a treatment; and to check for side-effects. Which tests are appropriate, if any at all, will depend on the individual and their type of arthritis.

Tests on blood samples are called haematology. When you give a sample ('Don't worry, you won't feel a thing'), it is usually placed in a series of tubes of different colours, each for a particular test. Happily they don't need to take too much – a pint of blood contains five thousand million white blood cells alone, so a syringeful is enough. Three types of blood cells are usually measured.

★ Red cells – these contain haemoglobin which carries oxygen around the body. A low haemoglobin level (called anaemia) may indicate a deficiency in iron or vitamins or, in rheumatoid arthritis, disease activity. In this case, monitoring haemoglobin levels helps monitor the disease; worsening anaemia may suggest a complication. People taking the more powerful antirheumatic drugs are regularly screened, because on rare occasions they may reduce the bone marrow cells which form blood. The ESR test measures the speed at which red blood cells settle under gravity. Inflammation increases the rate of settlement: the quicker the rate, the higher the ESR. A high ESR may, alongside other factors, suggest that your arthritis is becoming more active and causing more inflammation. The CRP test, which monitors levels of the protein CRP in the blood, also helps monitor inflammation.

★ White cells – these play a key defensive role in the body's immune system, multiplying swiftly to repel foreign invaders. (There is more about the immune system on page 53.) A rise in their numbers indicates an infection or, because of the increased autoimmune activity involved in these conditions, rheumatoid arthritis, lupus or similar. The doctor can learn more from closer examination of the three types of white cells (polymorphs, macrophages and lymphocytes) – a rise in one, perhaps, and not the others. A reduced lymphocyte count, for example, is typical of lupus. Drugs can also reduce the number of white cells, and this is why you may, if on certain stronger drugs, be required to take a monthly blood test.

★ Platelets, essential for blood-clotting, are also measured as they too can be reduced by certain drugs.

PHYSIOTHERAPISTS

You may be referred to a physio directly by your GP or through your consultant. Large general practices may have a resident or visiting physiotherapist or you may need to attend the local hospital. For physiotherapy, it is extremely unlikely that you will be referred to any hospital other than your local one.

Like GPs, hospital physios are generalists rather than specialists, so you may or may not get one with particular knowledge of your condition. If you have one of the more common forms of arthritis with fairly 'typical' mobility problems you should be fine. If not, it may be a bit of a lottery.

Physios are often crucial in the treatment of arthritis. They concentrate on relieving pain and improving mobility of the joints. They use manipulation and treatments such as ultrasound (which stimulates the body tissue using inaudible, high frequency sound waves), ice-packs and heat. They may well also show you exercises to do at home.

A typical course of treatment will last about ten sessions. Most hospitals are reluctant to provide anything that smacks of long-term care for financial reasons. If you have a long-term condition such as arthritis, this is not always helpful.

In some areas, you may be able to try hydrotherapy. This is a bit like physio in the water – although you won't have to lie on the couch! A hydrotherapy pool is specially heated but you may also be able to do the exercises you learn in the local swimming pool. (For more on exercising in water see page 125.)

Physiotherapy is also available privately. You may want to consider this if you feel you need more treatment than your hospital can provide, or if you need particularly specialised help. For names of local private physios, contact the Chartered Society of Physiotherapy who have a directory.

OCCUPATIONAL THERAPISTS (OT)

An OT will discuss your day-to-day activities both at home and work, and how they might be adapted to suit you. They can also advise on any aids or gadgets that might help, or even suggest structural alterations.

There are two very good reasons for thinking about how you approach your everyday activities. You want to make them as easy as possible, but you also want to protect your joints while doing them. Simply rearranging your home or adjusting the way you grip or lift something may make a real difference – and at no cost. (More about arthritis in the home and at work in Chapter 11.)

Your GP or consultant may refer you to an OT, or you can contact one yourself through your local council's Social Services department.

HOSPITAL SURGEONS

For some people with arthritis, surgery is suggested by their doctor. Operations for people with arthritis include joint replacement, joint fusion, removal of inflamed tissue, removal of some bone to ease pain, repair of damage to tendons, or relief of a trapped nerve.

Replacements are usually offered if the joint has become very badly damaged and is not responding to anything else. The most common is a hip replacement, although knees, ankles, shoulders, elbows and joints in the wrists and fingers can also be replaced. Put simply, the joint is removed under anaesthetic and replaced with an artificial one, called a prosthesis, made from plastic and metal.

Over 40,000 hips are replaced every year in this country. The operation's success rate is very high and a modern prosthesis can last fifteen years or more. With time, your range of joint movement should be about 75% of 'normal' and there is a 95% chance the operation will leave you pain-free. Knees are the second most commonly replaced joint.

If you have arthritis, it is not inevitable that at some point surgery will be needed – far from it. It is because it is relatively uncommon that the subject is not covered in detail in this short book.

If your doctor suggests a replacement operation, discuss what is being offered and why. How will it benefit you? The risks are small but you should ask about them. They include infection, thrombosis, dislocation of the joint and, in a very tiny number of cases, death. How will the new joint alter your lifestyle? What will you be able to do? What will you not be able to do? It is always your choice whether to proceed.

It is well worth trying to speak to other people who have experienced the operation or telephoning the Arthritis Care helpline. They can provide an information sheet or booklet as well as useful advice about how best to prepare for and recover from the operation.

Ian Loynes has had six successful replacement operations. 'I'm self-employed and need to maintain a fairly active lifestyle, so pain-free mobility is important. I'm lucky to have a good relationship with both my consultant and surgeon. Over the years we've conducted a plan of replacing joints as and when they get past an acceptable level of pain. My "pain-control" programme may seem very radical, and I sometimes wonder if I'm more artificial than real! But at the moment this "solution" gives the best result from the available options. For me, the small risk of a new joint failure is far outweighed by the pain-free result.'

The Patients' Charter guarantees a maximum wait for a hip or knee operation of eighteen months.

Marianne Rigge, the director of the College of Health, writing in *Which? Way to Health* magazine, says there are good and bad surgeons. The Royal Surgical Colleges of Great Britain and Ireland point out that 'a surgeon who performs a specific operation once or twice a year is unlikely to be as experienced, and therefore as competent, as a surgeon who performs the same procedure thirty times'.

Performance is monitored, but the information is not published. Marianne Rigge's organisation is campaigning for this. In the mean time she suggests talking to other patients, friendly doctors, the theatre sister or the relevant business manager within the hospital (who should be particularly keen to help if you have a fund-holding GP).

There are two commercial publications which may help. The entries in *The Medical Directory* are written by the doctors themselves, but do indicate their clinical interests, publications and membership of specialist organisations, while *The Good Doctor Guide* includes comments on doctors' reputations. Marianne Rigge says it is 'unofficial but well worth consulting'.

The College of Health runs the National Waiting-List Helpline.

COMMUNITY CARE

If, as a result of age, disability or illness, you need assistance in order to live your day-to-day life in your own home, you may be entitled to assistance under Community Care.

Community Care is arranged through your local Social Services department. You may be able to get help with the following: home help (such as cooking, shopping or more personal tasks such as dressing), meals on wheels, aids and equipment (a hand-rail for the bath, for example), counselling, occupational therapy and help with holidays, transport or installing a telephone.

To enable Social Services to determine your 'needs', the first step is an 'assessment'. Make an appointment with your Social Services department. In most parts of England and Wales, Social Services comes under the county council, although in London it is the borough council and, in bigger towns, the city or metropolitan council. In Scotland, social work comes under the regional council, in Northern Ireland under the local Health and Social Services Board or Trust.

Social Services are obliged to assess anyone who may need assistance under the relevant act (the NHS and Community Care Act 1993). The assessment interview will take place in your home or in a council office. You can have someone with you if you wish. The purpose of the assessment is to find out what needs you think you have, so make sure that you tell them. You could write down your needs and give the interviewer a copy. An assessment is free.

Most councils charge for the Community Care services they provide, although this charge should be reasonable – it should not be more than it costs the council to provide the service. Your interviewer will therefore ask questions about your ability to pay for any services you receive.

After the interview the interviewer should put your needs in writing and give you a copy. Social Services will then tell you which services they can offer to meet those needs. You may not get or be entitled to all the services you want. Equally, you can turn down any you don't want.

Voluntary organisations and local councils are monitoring Community Care very carefully. It would be misleading to suggest that there have not been problems with it since it was introduced in April 1993. How far these can be put down to 'teething troubles' is debatable. On the face of it, a policy which allows people to live in their own homes rather than institutions is to be welcomed, but the motives behind it continue to be questioned. Some say it is more about saving money.

Certainly there are many needs to be met and resourcing is a problem. A monitoring project by the voluntary organisation RADAR has shown that some local authorities are not yet satisfying the legal requirements of the 1970 Chronically Sick and Disabled Persons Act, let alone the 1990 NHS and Community Care Act. In one year RADAR had over 500 complaints from people whose Social Services departments were not meeting their statutory obligations. However, if you do need help in order to live in the community, you have nothing to lose by applying for Community Care. It is your right.

GETTING THE BEST OUT OF YOUR HEALTH PROFESSIONALS

It's your right to see a doctor and it's his or her job to treat you. However, if that's your attitude when you enter the surgery, you probably won't get as much out of your appointment as you would like. Like all human relationships, yours with your doctor needs working on if it's to be successful. It's strange. Most doctors are intelligent people who have entered their profession for the best of reasons. They've studied for years and they genuinely want to help you and everybody else who comes to see them. So why are they so difficult to talk to?

Partly it's down to us. It's embarrassing to talk about problems with your body with a complete stranger. What's more we don't feel in control, things are happening which we don't understand. We feel ignorant and scared: emotions that we are generally encouraged to repress or not to show.

Partly it's down to them. Doctors know an awful lot about the human body and how to keep it healthy, but you don't have to delve very far into the mysteries of medicine to discover how much they don't know. As we have seen, arthritis is a particularly complex disease. Even the specialist rheumatologist doesn't know all the answers (or even all the questions). Think about how the GP, who's had far less training, feels. Like you, they may feel a bit scared too – they are worried that they may be unable to help you.

They know that you will be expecting them to do something – that, after all, is why people go to see their doctor. We want treatment, relief, an explanation or answer. For any number of reasons, the doctor may not be able to give it. Especially not to someone appearing for the first time with joint pain. Arthritis can take a long time to diagnose.

One way for the doctor to deal with this is to adopt a more impersonal approach. Doctors' medical training can encourage this attitude. The body is divided up into sections like a motor car (making going to the chiropodist's a little like going down the tyre centre), and doctors learn to treat symptoms and diseases rather than people. Some complementary therapists, particularly those with their roots in eastern medicine, have criticised this approach for not being 'holistic', for not treating the whole person.

All this can make the doctor seem aloof, stand-offish, disinterested. If we stand back it all makes sense. Theoretically, we don't want our doctors to 'get involved'. We want them to deal objectively not emotionally with our problems. We don't want them to say things just to make us feel better. We want the truth. Theoretically. But when it's us sitting in that chair on the other side of the desk, well, if only they were a little more human.

The incredible thing is: they are. I toddled down the surgery the other day hoping to see my GP but I couldn't because she was off sick!

Don't put your doctor on a pedestal. Try to talk to them as you would a genuine friend. Even if at first they may not feel like one.

Don't trivialise how you feel or worry about wasting the doctor's time. Be honest about how you feel and about your pain – this can be particularly difficult for men.

It is not unreasonable to expect your doctor to speak to you in terms you can understand. If they do not, ask for an explanation: 'What do you mean by an antibiotic?'

In her excellent book, *Arthritis at Your Age*, Jill Holroyd suggests using an easy-to-understand yardstick for pain, grading it from one to ten, for example, where one is minor and ten unbearable. She also talks about pain with her doctor in terms of noise where the scale is from a whisper to a scream.

Make notes. Your doctor does and your doctor's a professional, so why shouldn't you? Beforehand, prepare answers to the questions that are regularly asked – how are you, for instance – and try to be as precise as possible: how painful? Where? When? Also list the questions you want to ask of your doctor and make sure you have time to ask them. If you are concerned about running out of time, let the doctor know: 'I've got three specific concerns I'd like to discuss before we finish.'

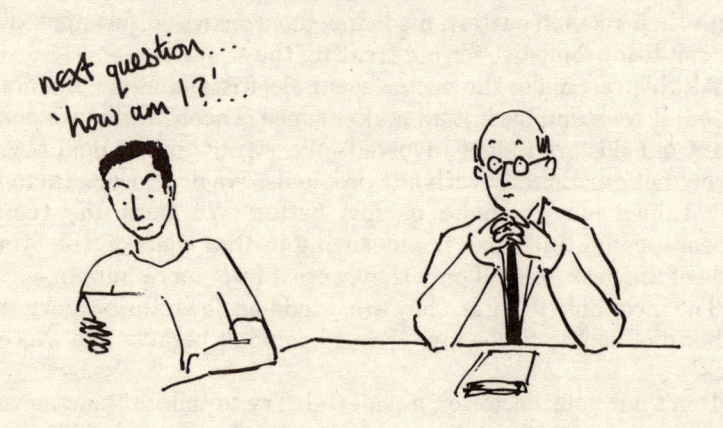

Try to be assertive. It can be very difficult when you are feeling bad and the doctor doesn't seem interested. However, you won't get another chance for a while. It's up to you to take this one. Ask for clarification: 'What do you mean by a couple more tests?' Ask for explanations: 'How much more exercise should I take? And what sort?' Being prepared and coming with notes will help.

Kate Lorig, an arthritis self-management trainer from America, believes that the good patient should be a CAD: 'Come prepared. Ask questions. Discuss problems.'

Afterwards make further notes. What did you discuss and what did you agree you would both do as a result? Did you say you'd try to lose some weight? How much? Did the doctor say they'd refer you to a physiotherapist? When will you hear? It makes sense to keep a notebook – a diary if you like – of all your medical appointments.

You could also use it to record how you feel between appointments, good days and bad days: when were they? What did they measure on the pain scale? Any ideas why?

These techniques can be applied equally well to your appointments with other health professionals. Before I started jotting things down I was more than capable of forgetting an exercise that the physio had shown me. I would then happily spend a week doing something completely irrelevant and possibly harmful.

By adopting some of these suggestions you may be able to improve your relationship with your doctor, but if you can't get along it is possible to change. The Patients' Charter says that you have the right to change your GP 'easily and quickly if you want to'. Contact your local Family Health Service Authority. They are expected to send you a full list of doctors within two working days, together with details of how to change doctors.

Doctors are busy professionals, so it helps if you take a professional approach too. They are also human beings who want to help you.

CHAPTER 5

Arthritis and Drugs

If you have arthritis, the chances are that your doctor will prescribe some drugs for you. In 1990, 23·3 million prescriptions for drugs to treat arthritis were dispensed – 5% of all NHS prescriptions – at a cost of £219 million. The charity Arthritis Care's membership survey suggests that four out of five people with arthritis are on prescribed drugs.

They're not miracle cures – they're just mixtures of chemicals which, when they mix with the chemicals in your body, are designed to do you some good. Sometimes doctors seem over-keen on prescribing drugs. Sometimes patients seem almost desperate to be given them. Try to take a considered approach. Discuss your medication with your doctor. An appointment does not have to end with the doctor presenting you with a freshly written prescription.

Drugs may be prescribed for a number of reasons: to relieve pain, to reduce inflammation or to suppress disease activity. In some cases they may be prescribed to offset the side-effects of other drugs. From coffee and alcohol to the most powerful anti-arthritis drug, all drugs can have side-effects. Some will be benign or harmless but some may be dangerous. Your doctor should always discuss with you the side-effects of any drug you are prescribed. If the doctor doesn't, you should ask. In the Arthritis Care survey, 46% of respondents had experienced unpleasant side-effects, mostly stomach pain.

Don't forget that over-the-counter drugs, that is, those you don't need a prescription for, have side-effects too.

The drugs industry

Drugs are big business. The UK market for prescription and non-prescription medicines was nearly £4·5 billion in 1992, of which sales to the NHS amounted to nearly £3·5 billion, almost 10% of total NHS expenditure. In total, 488 million items were issued on prescription.

The 1990s has seen prescriptions grow at a rate of about 4% a year compared to 2% in the previous two decades. This is largely because of the increasing number of elderly people.

Drug companies make and spend a lot of money. Because they make a lot of money some people question their priorities – patients or profit? The pharmaceutical industry argues that they need to make so much because they spend so much on researching and developing new drugs – £1·5 billion was spent in this way in 1992.

If you are one of those people who looks at the size and profits of the drug companies and gets a bit cynical, you're in good company. Dr Vernon Coleman, a well-known TV doctor and author of nearly fifty books, says in *How to Conquer Arthritis*: 'Worst of all, there seems to be a conspiracy between doctors and drug companies which ensures that millions of patients in pain are denied easy, cheap, reliable pain relief so that profits can remain.'

He's not joking, and he may have a point. The cheap, easy pain relievers he talks about, by the way, are those things you can do for yourself and which we'll talk about in much more detail later in this book. Coleman's world is the media now rather than medicine, so he's free to make comments which others may not be able to make.

Nevertheless, for the average little drug, it's a long, winding and expensive road to the shelves of your local pharmacist. All drugs must obtain a product licence from the Medicines Control Agency, who check that the research and trials have been conducted to a sufficient standard. The licence also indicates how the product may be used. Medicines are divided into three categories:

★ Prescription-only medicine – must be prescribed by a doctor or dentist and supplied by a pharmacist.

★ Pharmacy medicines – can be bought over the counter in a pharmacists (such as stronger painkillers like Nurofen).
★ General sales list (GSL) – can be bought in supermarkets and pretty much anywhere (such as paracetamol and aspirin). Buying drugs by their generic names (such as paracetamol or aspirin) is cheaper than buying them by their more familiar, TV-advertised brand names (such as Panadol or Anadin).

Current research is moving on from the approaches outlined in the rest of this section towards looking at the defects in the immune system which may cause rheumatoid arthritis. This is a long-term project. The Association of the British Pharmaceutical Industry says: 'It will be the next century before we know whether today's approaches are successful.' This means that if you read in the press of a 'new breakthrough in arthritis treatment', it should be taken with a pinch of salt.

The immune system
Many forms of arthritis, such as rheumatoid arthritis and systemic lupus erythamatosus, are autoimmune diseases. There are three main points which need to be understood.

★ The immune system is complex; one slight malfunction disturbs all the other parts. It is this complexity and the interrelation of all the parts which makes it difficult to devise treatments which act on the immune system.
★ The immune system shoots first and asks questions later. It is usually quiet, but when it detects a foreign invader in the body it multiplies at a rapid rate. Cells divide, providing a formidable army to repel the invasion. It is this feature that can make autoimmune diseases so serious. It is also the reason why so many drugs originally developed to fight cancer (in which cells also rapidly divide and multiply) are now used in arthritis.
★ Attacks in the immune system cause inflammation – the result of an immune attack is inflammation. Inflammation increases blood flow (causing heat and redness), makes the blood capillaries

leaky (causing swelling) and stimulates the nerve endings (causing pain).

Inflammation is a good thing when the immune system is working as it should: the successful repulsion of a bacterial invader through the skin, for example, will result in a boil. When the immune system turns on itself as in autoimmune diseases, arthritis can be the result.

Many of the drugs used to treat arthritis are anti-inflammatories. One of the central mediators of inflammation in rheumatoid arthritis is called tumour necrosis factor (TNF), and this is a focus for much research.

The major types of drugs
The next section looks at the major drugs used in the treatment of arthritis. For more information, the voluntary organisation Arthritis Care produces a series of easy-to-read drug sheets covering all the major drugs used in the treatment of arthritis.

ANALGESICS

Analgesics are painkillers. Those available over the counter, such as paracetamol, are non-narcotic. Paracetamol acts outside the brain but, in some way, inhibits perception of pain. Side-effects are unusual, but it is dangerous to exceed the stated dose.

Some drugs prescribed as analgesics are actually anti-inflammatories, such as aspirin and ibuprofen used in lower doses. See the section below on NSAIDs for a full explanation.

The narcotic analgesics are only available on prescription. They include morphine, buprenorphine, codeine, diamorphine, dihydrocodeine and pethidine. You may also encounter combination analgesics, combining a narcotic and a non-narcotic. Co-codamol, for example, contains paracetamol and codeine. If you are taking these you again need to check that you don't exceed the maximum dose of paracetamol – particularly if you are using straight paracetamol too. Be careful.

Narcotics work by mimicking the action of the body's natural painkillers called endorphins. They block the transmission of pain within the brain. Narcotics can make you feel sick, tired and constipated and occasionally make breathing difficult. Long-term use produces what doctors call 'tolerance' – in other words, you need a bigger dose to get the same effect. This obviously increases the risk of any side-effects.

Alcohol should be avoided with all analgesics.

NSAIDS

Non-steroidal anti-inflammatory drugs, or NSAIDs, are the most commonly prescribed anti-arthritis drugs. Twenty million prescriptions are written every year. Not surprisingly every drug company wants an NSAID or three. There are umpteen of them, and the mixture of generic (chemical) names and brand names can be very confusing. The one advantage of this to the patient is that if one NSAID doesn't work for you, there are plenty more to try.

Aspirin was the first NSAID, and a doctor once joked to me that the other NSAIDs are simply Newer Sorts of Aspirin In Disguise.

NSAIDs are analgesic, but their main use in arthritis is to reduce inflammation. They do this by blocking the production of prostaglandins, one of the 'chemical messengers' that the immune system uses to maintain inflammation. NSAIDs usually need to be taken for some time (as long as four weeks in some cases) before there is enough in the bloodstream to have any effect. As the body produces prostaglandins constantly, the benefits of NSAIDs are short-lived once you stop taking them.

Prostaglandins are also involved in other bodily functions, notably protecting the stomach and elsewhere from ulcers. It is because the prostaglandins also stop doing this job that gastrointestinal problems can develop with long-term NSAID use. Exactly what the problems are and how frequently they occur is still unclear. What is certain is that the safest NSAID is ibuprofen. Moderately safe NSAIDs include diclofenac, naproxen and indomethacin.

Because of these risks, you might be prescribed an anti-ulcer drug to use in tandem with your NSAID. The stomach needs to be protected from the acids and enzymes within it that break down food. Prostaglandins do this by helping in the production of mucus on the stomach lining. Without a thick layer of mucus, ulcers can form. If an ulcer forms near an artery more severe bleeding can result which may require hospital treatment – the risk is about 1% in a full year on the drug. Fatalities as a result of this are extremely rare.

Common cures for ulcers are cimetidine (brand name: Tagamet) and rantidine (Zantac). There are also single drugs such as Arthrotec with an NSAID centre and an anti-ulcer drug around it.

Long-term users of NSAIDs are advised to have regular blood tests to check for anaemia. Rarely, liver, kidney and skin reactions occur.

NSAIDs should be avoided by people with asthma and by women both in the first three months of pregnancy and at delivery. Use with caution if breast-feeding.

Some NSAIDs can also be applied topically – that is, directly on to the skin as creams. Although safer, they are not effective in all cases. Ask your doctor if they might work for you.

Common NSAIDs

Brand name	**Generic name**
Indocid	Indomethacin
Naprosyn	Naproxen
Brufen/Nurofen	Ibuprofen
Lederfen	Fenbufen
Feldene	Piroxicam
Voltarol	Diclofenac

DMARDS

DMARDs stands for disease-modifying anti-rheumatic drugs. This is rather a grand claim, since nobody really knows how

Arthritis and Drugs

DMARDs work. In rheumatoid arthritis they certainly don't appear to interfere with the actual disease process. SMARDs – symptom-modifying anti-rheumatic drugs – would probably be a better name.

If a doctor suspects your inflammatory arthritis (such as RA or lupus) may become more severe, he or she may well use these drugs fairly early on in your treatment. This is because most joint damage from arthritis occurs in the first two or three years. These are the main DMARDs:

★ Gold injections – given once a week in the buttock. Dosage: from 5–10mg initially, up to 50mg. Generic name: sodium aurothiomalate. Brand name: Myocrisin.
★ Oral Gold – better tolerated than gold injections but less effective. Dosage: usually 6mg a day, perhaps 9mg. Generic name: auranofin. Brand name: Ridaura.
★ Penicillamine – taken one hour before or after food. Iron tablets should not be taken within an hour and a half of taking penicillamine. Dosage: from 125mg a day initially, up to 250–500mg. Brand names: Distamine or Pendramine.
★ EC-Sulphasalazine – taken with water after food. Plenty of water should be drunk to avoid any kidney reaction. EC means enteric-coated. This special coating lets the tablets pass through the stomach before releasing their contents. Dosage: from 500mg a day initially, up to 2,000–3,000mg. Brand name: Salazopyrin-EN.

Side-effects of DMARDs include nausea, diarrhoea, skin rashes and mouth ulcers. Gold, penicillamine and sulphasalazine can reduce production of red blood cells in the bone marrow, so a regular blood test is required. Urine tests are also used with gold and penicillamine because of the possibility of kidney damage. When taking sulphasalazine your urine may become orange, but this is nothing to worry about. Occasionally you may, when starting penicillamine, lose your sense of taste. This will return after six weeks or so whether or not you are still taking the drug. Ringing in the ears (called tinnitus) has been reported with sulphasalazine. Tell your doctor about any side-effect. Moderate alcohol consumption is safe with DMARDs.

ANTI-MALARIAL DRUGS

Hydroxychloroquin (brand name: Plaquenil) and chloroquine (Avloclor), originally used in the treatment of malaria, are often used in the treatment of lupus and sometimes in rheumatoid arthritis. They are usually taken with food once or twice daily. The safe dose is less than 6·5mg per kilo of your ideal (rather than actual) body weight. An ideal body weight chart is on pages 94–5.

The major side-effect is possible damage to the retina of the eye. For this reason you will need a regular eye test and may be given a piece of paper with lines on it (called an Amsler grid) to check your own sight with. Other side-effects include stomach upsets, disturbed sleep, skin rashes, dizziness and headaches.

IMMUNOSUPPRESSORS

Immunosuppressors are slow-acting and do not tackle pain or inflammation directly. NSAIDs or analgesics will be prescribed for use alongside. Immunosuppressors might also be used in order to minimise doses of steroids (see next section).

Cyclophosphamide (brand name: Endoxana) and methotrexate (Emtextate or Matrex) were originally developed to prevent cancer cells growing and dividing. At lower doses they can be used to counter the rapid cell division that occurs in auto-immune diseases such as rheumatoid arthritis or lupus.

Methotrexate is generally taken following your evening meal. Folic acid may be prescribed if you feel sick afterwards. The dose begins low (around 2·5mg) and rises to 7·5–20mg.

Cyclophosphamide is usually taken as a tablet in the morning with food although in hospital it may be given intravenously.

Other immunosuppressors, such as Cyclosporin A (Sandimmum) and azathioprine (Azamune or Imuran), were first produced to prevent rejection in transplant operations. Azathioprine is taken once or twice a day after food in doses up to 2·5mg per kilo of body weight.

Side-effects of immunosuppressors: because they act on the immune system, immunosuppressors can reduce resistance to infectious disease. As with DMARDs, they can also reduce red cell production and, again, blood tests should be given regularly.

Methotrexate can cause skin rashes, ulcers or soreness in the mouth, vomiting and diarrhoea. It can also react with alcohol making drinking inadvisable. Cyclophosphamide can cause haemorrhagic cystitis, which makes passing water painful and blood appear in the urine. Drinking lots of water can minimise this risk. Cyclophosphamide can also cause hair loss and irregular periods.

Both can affect fertility. Women should stop taking either methotrexate or cyclophosphamide several months before trying to conceive. Men should stop methotrexate six months before trying while cyclophosphamide, if you are thinking of ever starting a family, is best avoided.

STEROIDS

Steroids have an important part to play in the body. They are 'chemical messengers'. Produced naturally by the adrenal glands in the kidneys, they travel around in the blood doing all sorts of useful jobs. One particular group, corticosteroids, are involved in the metabolism (breaking down) of food and affect the balance of water and salt in the body. However, it is because they are also involved in regulating inflammation and our immune systems that they can be used to treat inflammatory diseases. Strictly speaking then, when people talk about the steroids used in the treatment of arthritis, they actually mean corticosteroids. These steroids are nothing like those used, often illegally, by some athletes and body-builders.

A synthetic version of corticosteroid is used and administered in rather higher doses than the body would naturally produce. It can be injected directly into the inflamed joint or used as a tablet to combat more general inflammation and suppress the immune system.

★ Injections – Giving an injection concentrates the steroid in the crucial area, reducing the chances of the side-effects that can occur with a tablet. First, the joint is cleaned with cotton wool and alcohol and, in some cases, fluid removed from the joint using a syringe. Then a small dose of steroid and local anaesthetic is injected. The joint should be rested for a day or so, however good it might feel! At the site of the injection, there may be a thinning in the fat beneath the skin and a loss of skin colour.

★ Tablets – Prednisolene is by far the major steroid taken by mouth (there are others which are injected), and it rejoices in a host of brand names: Cortisol, Deltacortril Enteric, Deltastab, Precortisyl, Prednesol and Sintisone. Generally, it is taken as one tablet in the morning after food. It is a powerful anti-inflammatory and reduces activity among the white blood cells. However, this power is difficult to target – corticosteroids go in all guns blazing – so side-effects are a big problem. It is generally used when all other treatments have failed or there are complications in the disease such as the involvement of major organs or the possibility of vasculitis (inflamed blood vessels).

Oral steroids take over from your natural source of corticosteroids, the adrenal glands, and so the body quickly becomes dependent on the tablets. This means oral steroids should never be stopped suddenly. The body needs to be weaned off them to allow the adrenal gland to start doing its job again. If you are taking steroids, carry a card (which your doctor should give you) or wear a medical information bracelet so that your dose can be continued should anything happen to you.

The side-effects from steroids are severe. You need to consider them carefully and discuss them with your doctor before embarking on a steroids programme. Equally, you need to be aware of the potential dangers from an untreated inflammatory disease.

Side-effects can include water retention, making you feel

bloated; muscle fatigue, from lost potassium; and the redistribution of weight from the arms and legs to the face and body. This, coupled with the water retention, can cause you to put on weight. Skin can become thin, bruise easily and become prone to rashes and acne. Calcium loss can lead to thinning of the bones and osteoporosis. On steroids, you can become more prone to illness and infection. High doses also affect blood pressure, moods and sleep. In extreme cases, steroids can cause heart failure.

For all these reasons, doses should be kept as low as possible. That is why steroids are often used in tandem with immunosuppressors or DMARDs. It is generally considered that at doses below 7·5mg per day, major side-effects are unlikely to occur. At this level the adrenal gland still has to do some work of its own. Sometimes your doctor might prescribe steroids every other day.

When corticosteroids were first developed in the fifties they were hailed as miracle drugs and the doctors involved awarded the Nobel Prize. However, it is now recognised that there is a price to pay for their power and doctors should use them with care.

HOW TO GET THE BEST OUT OF DRUGS

When your doctor prescribes drugs for you, make sure you know exactly what they are. If you are keeping a journal of pain and other symptoms, exercise and activities and so on, to help you prepare for your doctor's appointments, why not record drug information here too? It can take time to find the right drug for you. Knowing exactly what you're taking will help you to assess the effects. You'll be able to weigh up the various alternatives (and remind the doctor which tablets you've already tried!).

Your pills check-list
Ask your doctor the following:

★ What's the drug called? Both the brand name and the generic.
★ How many should you take and how often? Before or after eating? At bedtime? What should you do if you miss a dose?

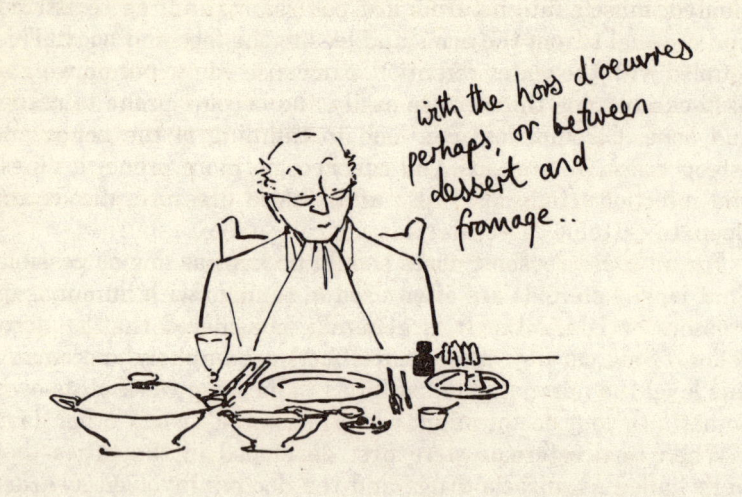

with the hors d'oeuvres perhaps, or between dessert and fromage...

★ What does it do? Is it a painkiller (analgesic), an anti-inflammatory, a disease modifier? What specific benefits should you feel?
★ How quickly will it work? Some drugs work more quickly than others.
★ How strong is it? In milligrams. It is important to know exactly how much of a drug you are taking.
★ What are the possible side-effects? Is there anything you can do to avoid them? What should you do if you suspect you may be experiencing them?
★ What should be avoided while taking the drug? Alcohol? Driving? Operating machines?

With certain drugs such as steroids where it is important that the course of treatment is not interrupted, you will be given an information card which should be carried at all times. With others, such as Gold, you should be issued with a record card to be filled in after every treatment, blood and urine test.

One point which isn't always stressed enough in the doctor's surgery is the importance of taking the drugs at the right time

Arthritis and Drugs

and in the right quantity. People use all sorts of methods to remind them: watch alarms, kitchen timers, notes in a diary, good-natured partners and so on. You can even buy a beeping pill box! For a balanced intake, take your drugs according to the clock and your doctor's instructions, not according to how much pain you feel. Lurching from one extreme to the other makes it harder to assess the medication and can be very disruptive to your everyday life.

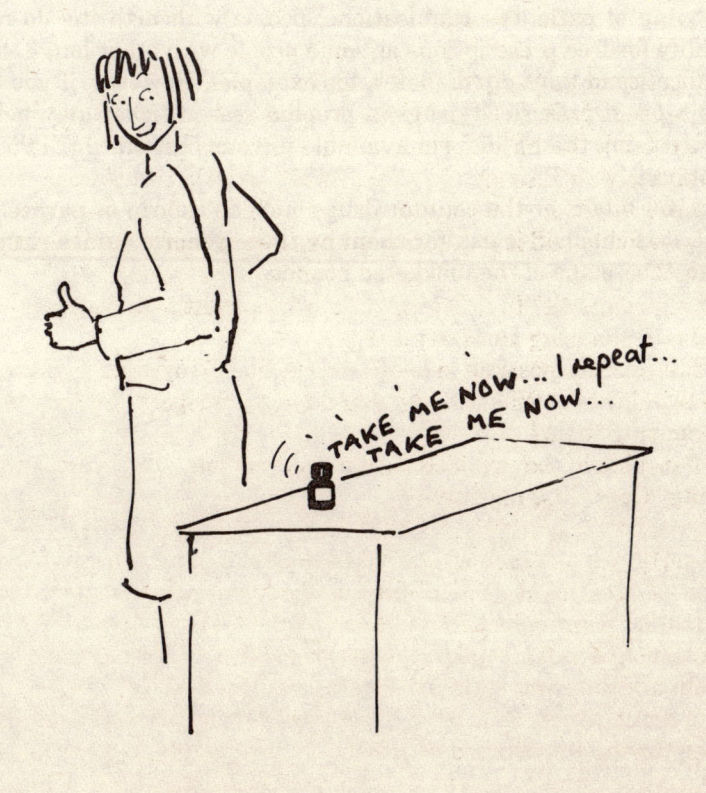

It helps your doctor to prescribe the right medication if you are blunt about how you feel. Being brave means you may get the wrong drug or a dose that is too low. There is evidence that too little of a painkiller is far more likely to lead to dependency than too much, because the body notices the difference it makes far more.

You should also be frank with your doctor about side-effects. With NSAIDs, for example, there are a number of strategies you can employ to reduce stomach pain: spreading the dose (more frequent doses of weaker tablets); changing the time at which the dose is taken (for example, the stomach lining is coated after eating); trying a coated tablet (which will pass through the stomach before releasing its contents); or taking an antacid alongside the drug. This advice also applies to any aspirin you might have bought over the counter.

Prescriptions are expensive. At the time of writing, they cost £5·25 an item and the charge tends to rise every year. Despite the lobbying of patients' organisations, people with arthritis do not qualify for free prescriptions as some people with other long-term medical conditions do (diabetes, for example). However, if you do use a lot of prescribed drugs, a prepaid season ticket may help. Apply using the FP95 form available in your post office (EP95 in Scotland).

If you buy over-the-counter drugs such as aspirin or paracetamol, it is cheaper to ask for them by these generic names rather than choose one of the marketed brands.

CHAPTER 6

Arthritis and Complementary Therapies

Once upon a time it was called alternative medicine; now it is more usually called complementary. Increasingly, doctors are realising that there is a role for other types of treatment to play alongside their own. It's just as well really, because thousands, probably millions of people with arthritis use them. Arthritis usually lasts a long time, and often doctors cannot offer as much for it as they and their patients would like. No wonder people look elsewhere. However, beware. This growth in interest can be exploited by unscrupulous practitioners. Before you explore the wide and interesting array of complementary therapies, make sure you are well informed.

For most people with arthritis treatment is under the NHS, using what is sometimes called 'conventional' medicine. The drugs used have been clinically tested in a particular way and are licensed for use by the Medicines Control Agency.

Complementary therapies have not been through the same regulatory process. Many see the body and good health in a very different way to conventional western science. The approach may not have been researched at all in the conventional way; evidence is often anecdotal, based on users' own experiences rather than laboratory research. However, do not let that put you off. It is not an exaggeration to say that complementary therapies have revolutionised the lives of some people with arthritis.

Complementary approaches do not divide the body into a series of separate units as western doctors can do. They take a holistic approach – treating the whole person. As the patient, you and your views are therefore at the centre of the process. (No wonder it's so popular). Complementary therapies also try to exploit the body's capacity to heal itself.

In 1991 a survey by the Consumers Association, who publish *Which?* magazine, found that one in four people had visited a complementary therapist in the previous year. If they did the survey again it would be one in three or even higher.

Doctors, too, are softening their attitude – the British Medical Association has now produced its first guide to complementary therapies. The most widely accepted therapies among GPs are acupuncture, osteopathy, chiropractic and hypnosis.

Your GP can refer you to an NHS medical homeopath and may be able to buy in services from an osteopath, chiropractor or acupuncturist. Some private medical insurers too will now pay out for complementary therapies.

To maintain professional standards, many therapies have their own regulatory body – sometimes, unfortunately, more than one – but practitioners do not have to join them. Under British law anyone can set up anywhere and call themselves pretty much anything they like – no training required. The various regulatory bodies are listed in Chapter 13 and you are well advised to check that your practitioner is a member. Osteopaths and chiropractors now have statutory bodies recognised by the Government.

Complementary therapies don't work for everybody and, arguably, some of them don't work for anybody. Most are time-consuming. Some are expensive and one or two of the more whacky fringe therapies may be harmful to some people. The various practitioners have theories as to how their particular therapies work, just as doctors do about the treatments they use, and these are covered under the appropriate section. In some cases it is fair to say that no one really knows. However, there are some general points worth bearing in mind.

★ The placebo effect – In drugs trials some people are given the drug under scrutiny and others are given something that looks exactly the same but does nothing. It's called a placebo. Many people on the placebo still get better. This goes to show the importance of your state of mind in healing. If you believe you're going to get better you're more likely to. Doctors often dismiss the successes of complementary approaches as the placebo effect. However, many people using them don't really care how they work for them. They're just happy that they do.

This difference of opinion reflects the different perspectives of doctor and patient. The doctor, as a scientist, wants to know why it works. The patient, as a person with arthritis, just wants to know if it works. Discuss what complementary medicine might do for you with your GP, try to see your doctor's point of view – but ultimately do what feels right for you.

★ The power principle – On the other side of the placebo coin is the power principle. Simply by trying something of your choice for yourself will make you feel more in control. And what's more, complementary approaches put you right at the centre of the treatment: you're the boss. Don't underestimate how good taking power can feel.

One of the people quoted in Andrew Vickers' invaluable little book *Complementary Medicine and Disability* captures the

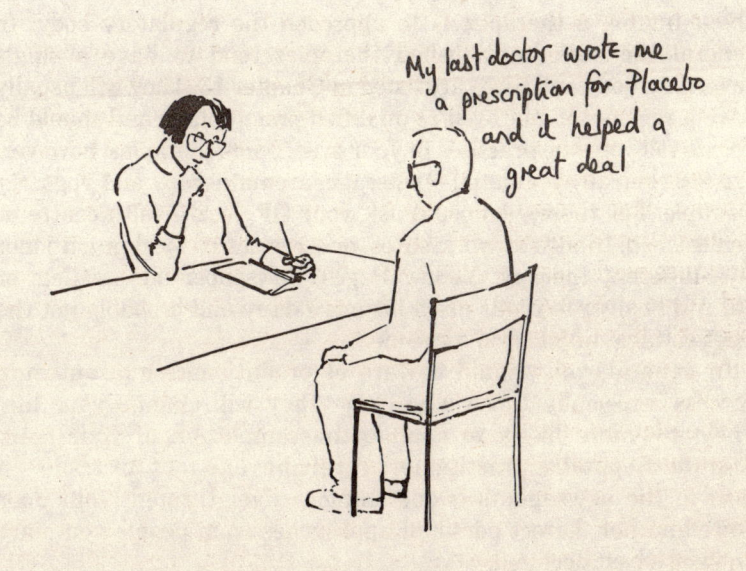

My last doctor wrote me a prescription for Placebo and it helped a great deal

difference between her doctor and her complementary therapist starkly and succinctly: 'Instead of banging on about "clinical this" and "clinical that" and using forty-eight-syllable words, she carefully explained to me what she was doing and why.' All the comments on the particular therapies in this chapter are from people with arthritis who have tried them.

HOW TO CHOOSE A THERAPIST

The first thing to do is decide which therapy you fancy. Systemic forms of arthritis such as rheumatoid arthritis and systemic lupus erythematosus are more likely to respond successfully to homeopathy, nutritional or herbal approaches than osteoarthritis. Osteopathy and chiropractic can ease stiff joints and increase mobility (although manipulative therapies should be avoided when joints are damaged or inflamed). Yoga can also aid mobility. Acupuncture is particularly good for pain relief.

Once you know which therapy you want to try, the best way to go about finding a therapist is to approach the regulatory body. In general the better established therapies tend to have a single governing body and these are listed in Chapter 13. They will usually have a register of approved or qualified practitioners and should be able to tell you who practises in your area. Some therapies, however, are not centrally regulated – massage, aromatherapy and yoga, for example. For these, you could ask your GP, local health centre or health shop, friends or workmates, or a registered local practitioner of a different therapy. Yellow Pages, newspaper ads, leaflets or natural healing festivals are a bit more dicey and probably not the most suitable way to find someone.

In general, you should beware of practitioners guaranteeing success, especially those who claim they will change your life. They are more likely to change the complexion of your bank account. Reputable practitioners rarely have to tout for trade – a card in the newsagents is one thing, a flyer through your door quite another. Direct personal approaches from people you don't know are best declined.

Check out the people you are considering. Ask what they do and how long they've been doing it. What training have they had, where and for how long? How did they become interested in the therapy? As a rule of thumb, Andrew Vickers says: 'The more a practitioner promises, the less they will be able to provide.'

Once you have chosen a therapist, you can always change your mind. Because of the person-centred approach of complementary therapies, it is essential that you feel comfortable with them. If your practitioner bullies you or attacks you personally for your lack of progress or inability to do what they suggest, forget them. No competent complementary therapist will behave like this.

To get anything out of the experience, it goes without saying that it is important that you understand what the therapist is saying. If you don't, the advice is the same as with your doctor: ask. If their talk is all mystical mumbo-jumbo more suited to children's fairy tales, they may be more interested in confusing you than treating you. You are paying; you have the right to practical help that is useful to you in your life.

This chapter covers the complementary therapies most popular with people with arthritis.

ACUPUNCTURE

The roots of this ancient therapy – acupuncture is at least 5,000 years old – can be found in China. It was unknown in the West before the Second World War and did not make much impression until President Nixon visited China and watched the technique being used.

For people with arthritis, it is most useful for pain relief. It cannot alter the actual disease process.

The theory of acupuncture is that good health depends on the flow of energy through the body – a balance between Yin (passive and cold) and Yang (hot and active). This flow can be adjusted or improved at specific points on the body, called acupoints, by the insertion of special needles. These points are located along twelve meridians joining various organs. By working on particular acupoints, the acupuncturist can treat the organs that share its meridian. Stimulating the acupoints with the fingers or a TENS machine (see below) can also help.

Acupuncturists may also burn a special herb, moxa, just above the skin. This is called moxibustion and is believed to nourish the Chi energy.

Western and Chinese medicine explain the success of acupuncture in different ways. Acupuncturists believe that the treatment promotes the flow of healing energy, known as Chi, along the meridians. Western physicians say the acupoints are on the nerve pathways and the needles prompt the body to release its own painkillers (called endorphins). Because it also appears to increase the natural corticosteroids (see section on steroids on page 59) in the body, acupuncture can be employed alongside drug treatment.

An initial consultation with an acupuncturist will cost £20–30 and last between half an hour and an hour and a half. The practitioner will take a medical history and will be particularly interested in how the time of year, time of day and weather affect you. Heat, cold, dryness, wind and damp can all affect your Chi. They will also examine your face and tongue and observe you walk, talk, sit and stand. Fine needles will then be inserted into the appropriate acupoints – usually these are on the arms and legs, hands and feet. Most people say that the needles do not hurt. They are barely thicker than a human hair and between two and six are usually used.

Subsequent consultations will be shorter and cost around £20. Up to six sessions may be required – perhaps more for a long-standing problem.

For more information contact The British Medical Acupuncture Society or The Council For Acupuncture.

Consumer's report
'I started acupuncture for a specific problem when I was very distraught and depressed. The specific problem has since been operated on, but my general well-being, my spirit, my attitude, my whole life has turned around. The only time it has ever hurt was when I was about to go down with the most nasty bout of flu.'

TENS machines

Transcutaneous Electrical Nerve Stimulation (TENS), which stimulates the acupoints through rubber electrodes, sounds like the modern hi-tech adaptation of acupuncture. However, a forerunner even for this can be found among the early civilisations: the Romans practised something similar with electric eels!

Today's TENS machines, a small box about the size of a personal stereo, are just as portable and don't wriggle around so much. Although you need to be shown how to use the machine by a specialist such as a physiotherapist, you can usually attach the electrodes and practise the treatment yourself although it can be fiddly. The electrodes are attached using adhesive tape or gel, and a low voltage current passed through them. This should be set, again with the initial help of a specialist, at a level just below that which is slightly painful for you.

TENS does not work for everyone. Their success rate is perhaps 50–60%. Some users have reported skin reactions to the gel and tape. The machines can also be quite expensive but you ought to be able to borrow one through the NHS. Ask your GP or physio. Arthritis Care can provide a fact sheet – send an SAE.

Consumer's report

'I used the machine for about two hours each day and found it helped to ease my pain a great deal. I usually used mine in the evening when I was able to sit down and relax. It didn't take the pain away completely but it did relieve it for a while. Some hospitals loan them out, and I'd suggest you try this first. Personally, I did find it most useful. Like anything, you don't know until you give it a go.'

Shiatsu

Shiatsu, which means finger pressure, began in Japan. It involves the manipulation with the fingers of the acupoints, called 'tsubo' in shiatsu. It shares acupuncture's philosophy of Chi and the meridians and so on, but with some variations in practice. A shiatsu practitioner will usually work over the whole body, tending to 'feel' what's going on rather than make a full diagnosis before treatment begins. For this reason, the initial discussion in shiatsu tends to be shorter than with many other complementary approaches.

Treatment is generally on a thick floor-mat rather than a couch, and usually takes place with your clothes on – wear something loose and light. The therapist will combine touching, stretching, rubbing and squeezing over the tsubo. It should not be painful.

Combining as it does aspects of massage with acupuncture, shiatsu brings some of the benefits of each. For people with arthritis, it can stimulate blood flow, ease stiff muscles and promote a feeling of well-being.

Sessions last from forty minutes to an hour and cost around £20–25. For more information contact The Shiatsu Society.

ALEXANDER TECHNIQUE

It's easy to fall into bad habits. But the bad habits actor F.M. Alexander found he had fallen into a hundred years ago were not drinking, smoking and luvvies' late nights but speaking, walking, sitting and standing.

Alexander became unable to perform because his voice continually failed him. With his doctors ineffective, he decided to try to sort the problem out for himself, spending hours in front of the mirror watching himself recite and perform simple movements. He retrained himself in these everyday activities and this is what Alexander Technique teachers do today. This involves, in Alexander's words, bridging 'the gap between the subconscious and the unconscious'.

The study of babies and animals suggests that we have naturally good posture and co-ordination in movement, but that this is interfered with as we get older. So Alexander teachers often encourage their pupils to enjoy a 'child-like' approach to movement.

Alexander lessons are generally one-to-one and, initially at least, two or even three lessons a week may be suggested.

Alexander's is not therefore a cheap technique to learn. Lessons usually cost between £15 and £25. Alexander reckoned that he could teach in four weeks what it took him ten years to learn. He tended to suggest daily lessons but today's Alexander teachers are more modest about its immediate benefits, tending to stress the longer-term effects.

Alexander Technique is considered particularly good for stress-related conditions including arthritis, head- and backache and for living with pain. Classes last about forty-five minutes and involve working on standing and sitting and lying in the basic Alexander semi-supine position: on your back on a table with the head supported by books, feet flat on the table and the knees bent, pointing towards the ceiling. The teacher will touch and draw attention to your joints but it is simply that: touching, not manipulation.

It is very difficult, even for teachers, to explain how the technique works or even what is involved. Stopping and thinking and allowing the body to find its natural balance plays an important role. However, if we are trying too hard, if we concentrate too much in our attempts to lengthen our muscles, we merely tighten and stiffen: the opposite of what is required. Alexander teachers encourage pupils to 'think the neck free in order to allow the head to go forward and up in order to allow the back to lengthen and widen'.

Pupils report greater lightness and freedom in movement and a more positive outlook on life. Although it is well-established and respected, with more than 500 teachers in the UK, doctors are only now beginning to prescribe it.

If you are interested in learning the Alexander Technique, the most important thing is to find a teacher you feel comfortable with. The Society of Teachers of the Alexander Technique (STAT) can help. All members have completed a three-year training course.

Consumer's report
'I have a lesson every seven to ten days and they are certainly relaxing. The most noticeable thing about AT is that nothing happens in any active sense. My teacher says that we have to

learn consciously to do movements and activities that normally we perform unconsciously. It's a tall order but fortunately that's how it usually makes me feel: a little taller. In the lying position, the teacher works all the way down one side of your body and then all the way down the other side: each muscle "unhooking" like a taut octopus clip. It's hard to believe that simply by wishing the neck free it can happen, but it seems to. The teacher's role is to suggest, to verbalise the wish and focus it.'

CHIROPRACTIC

Joint manipulation as a form of medicine is considerably younger than say acupuncture – barely 2,000 years old. Chiropractic as practised today began in Canada a century ago.

In this country it is one of the most widely respected complementary therapies. Its regulatory body, The British Chiropractic Association, was established as long ago as 1925, and a 1994 act passed in parliament will set up an approved register of chiropractors.

Its originator, Canadian Daniel David Palmer, saw the spine as quite literally central to physical well-being. The spine houses the central nervous system so, if the spine's mobility is impeded, the nervous system may be affected and problems occur in other parts of the body.

The chiropractor examines the spine for joints whose movement has become limited. These are called 'fixations'. They may have been caused by an injury, allergy, lack of nutrition, stress or posture. Treatment essentially involves moving the joint surfaces apart and getting them moving again. This takes place on a treatment couch.

For people with arthritis, chiropractic may ease stiff muscles and joints and increase mobility. The treatment is particularly successful with pain in the lower back, upper body, head and neck.

It is best avoided if there is inflammation in the spine, during a flare-up or if you may have osteoporosis. Indeed, if you are thinking about chiropractic or any other manipulative therapy such as osteopathy, it is particularly important to discuss it with your GP. Practised on the wrong person in the wrong way they can be dangerous.

When you first visit a chiropractor, you will be asked a wide range of questions about your lifestyle. X-Rays may be taken. The chiropractor will then observe how you use your muscles and spine when walking, standing, leaning over and so on. You will need to undress down to your underwear for this. The initial assessment takes around half an hour and costs about £35. Subsequent visits, costing £20–30, take about fifteen minutes.

For further information contact The British Chiropractic Association.

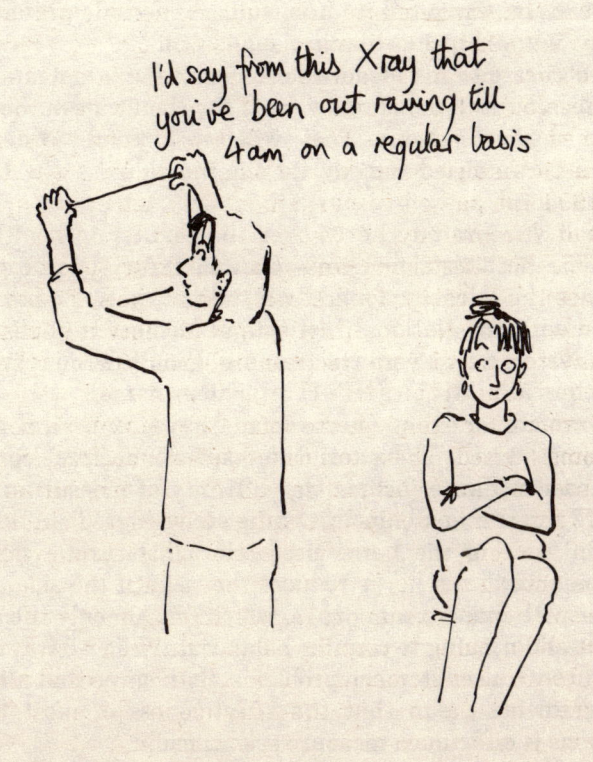

I'd say from this Xray that you've been out raving till 4am on a regular basis

HERBAL MEDICINE

Another therapy with an ancient Eastern tradition. Records of medicinal herbs found in northern China have been carbon-dated to 3000 BC. Herbal medicine also has a fine pedigree in the West – many drugs are based on herbal remedies. Aspirin, for example, includes a substance found in the bark of the willow tree.

In fact, most cultures have developed their own herbal remedies. The Chinese type is founded in the same theory of Yin and Yang and the flow of Chi as acupuncture. Herbalists use herbs to maintain these balances.

In England there is also a tradition of herbal healing. The idea is that by cleaning and rebalancing the body, its natural healing process can be exploited to the full. A herbal 'prescription' therefore may well include dietary suggestions.

It is inaccurate to see modern herbalism as an amalgam of old wives' tales. Practitioners are aware of the chemicals in the herbs and their medical actions. They will try to combine herbs to produce a personalised remedy for the individual – the holistic approach again.

Although you can buy herbs over the counter in health food shops, some herbalists feel this mix-and-match DIY approach undermines the scientific foundation to their craft. Practitioners registered with the National Institute of Medical Herbalism, for example, undergo four years of training. (You can identify them by the letters MNIMH or FNIMH after their name.)

While accepting that herbs can have anti-viral, anti-inflammatory and anti-bacterial properties, doctors' concerns about herbal medicine include the difficulty of measuring doses accurately and the small amount of the active ingredient actually present in some of the herbs used. Herbalists argue that the natural balance of the herbs reduces the risks of the side-effects that occur with mainstream drugs, which contain only the active ingredient and nothing to counter-balance it. Willow bark, unlike aspirin, rarely causes stomach problems. Both agree that all these other ingredients mean that the effectiveness of most herbal preparations is difficult to measure scientifically.

Arthritis and Complementary Therapies

The first visit costs around £25 (plus the price of anything prescribed). You will be asked for a full medical and dietary history and be examined. Some tests may be carried out.

If you have arthritis, you will not necessarily be prescribed an anti-inflammatory. Other problems, like constipation, may be targeted first. Herbal medicine is particularly good with digestion and elimination problems. These, if treated, may lead to improvements in your joints.

You may be given ointments, poultices (a hot, moist application for the skin – from the Latin for porridge!), syrups (where the herb has been boiled in water with sugar) or tinctures (including alcohol). Most herbs are slow-acting, so give them time.

Unless you have problems with your prescription or it doesn't appear to be working, a single visit to the herbalist may be sufficient.

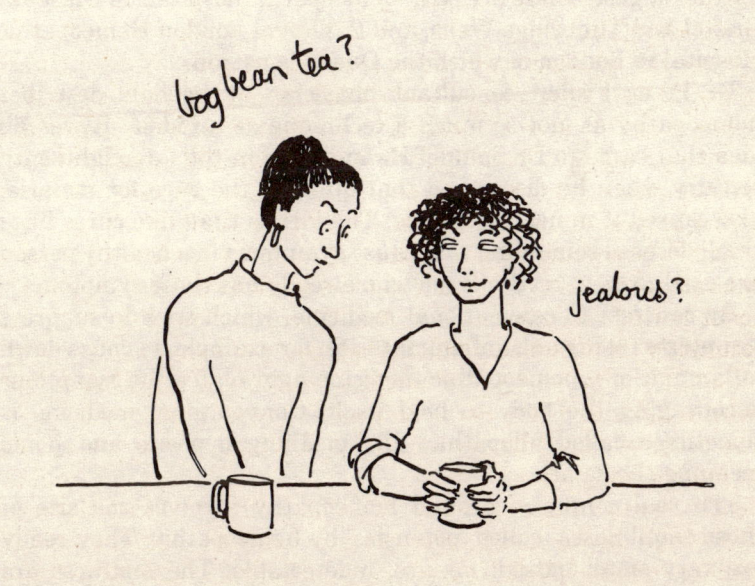

Lida Clark, who studied for five years at the National Institute of Herbal Medicine and is now a counsellor for people with arthritis, recommends three small cups of celery seed or bog bean tea a day as diuretics (that is, they make it easier to pee!). She says, 'The diuretic action is useful since it aids the body in getting rid of excess fluid, which can build up around the joints and cause painful pressure.'

You could also try a small cup of wild thyme tea a day. 'It has anti-bacterial properties as well as helping digestion, aiding healing and inducing a calmer state of mind.' These herbs should be available in good health food shops or reputable herbalists. Use the standard infusion indicated on the packet.

For further information contact the National Institute of Herbal Medicine.

HOMEOPATHY

Although nobody really understands how homeopathy works, it is the complementary therapy that has been available on the NHS for the longest. There are NHS homeopathic hospitals in Glasgow, Bristol and Tunbridge Wells, and the Royal London Homeopathic Hospital in London of which the Queen is patron.

Dr Peter Fisher, consultant physician at London, describes homeopathy as 'not so much a technique as an idea'. It was an idea that came to Dr Samuel Hahnemann in the late eighteenth century when he discovered that quinine, the cure for malaria, also caused it in healthy people. The idea is that 'like cures like': small doses of something that cause symptoms in a healthy person are used to treat an ill person who already has those symptoms.

By contrast to conventional medicine, which tries to suppress symptoms (using anti-inflammatories, for example, to douse down inflammation), homeopathic medicine aggravates the symptoms encouraging the body to heal itself. Conventional medicine is sometimes called allopathic: allo meaning opposite and homo meaning the same.

The real confusion around homeopathy involves the size of those small doses (called 'potencies' by homeopaths). They really are very small indeed: minute, indetectable. The mixtures are diluted in water time and time and time again until the original molecules of the 'active ingredient' have, according to the laws of physics, diluted away. So how can it work if there is nothing there? Homeopaths believe that it leaves behind an imprint of the original molecules' energy – the so-called 'memory of water'. Not surprisingly, this is very controversial. The only study that came anywhere near to showing this scientifically was riddled with errors and has never been repeated.

A comprehensive overview of all the tests and trials of homeopathic medicine was undertaken in Holland in 1991. No trial showed how it worked – the researchers said the 'memory of water' theory would mean that 'essential concepts of modern physics would have to be dismissed' – but the balance of trials showed that it did work. They looked at 107 trials altogether and, although some were of dubious scientific validity, eighty-one produced results favourable to homeopathy.

Because homeopathy works by adjusting the body's own healing mechanisms, it works best in forms of arthritis where there is active disease. The best results occur early on before joints become damaged. Homeopathic medicine cannot reverse what's already been done, although it may slow down further progression. It is also less effective in non-inflammatory disease or once inflammatory disease has burned out.

The holistic principle is central to homeopathy – practitioners treat people, not diseases. Dr Fisher says it 'can often make patients feel stronger and better in themselves, even when the disease is advanced'. This, while it is grist to the mill for those who want to dismiss homeopathy as the placebo effect writ large, is good news for you, the patient.

The first visit to a homeopath will involve a detailed medical and personal history, including your diet and any recent causes of stress such as a bereavement or other domestic or work difficulty. The homeopath will try to build up a picture of what is known as your constitutional type: your physical and emotional state. This will help determine the appropriate remedy for you. You could call it a 'horses for courses' approach. Dr Fisher prefers to explain it in terms of seed and soil: 'The seeds of a particular disease can only flourish in the soil of certain kinds of people.' This customised approach to treatment means that if you are seriously interested in homeopathy it is important to see a qualified practitioner rather than dabbling too much in DIY.

The homeopath will also try to pin down very accurately exactly what you want treated: pain, stiffness, in which joints and so on. This is because only one homeopathic remedy is used at a time.

If you see a homeopath privately, this initial consultation will last up to one and a half hours and cost £20–30. Follow-up sessions may be shorter but the homeopath will still ask all about how the treatment is going. There are two types of homeopath: medical ones who have also had a doctor's training and non-medical ones who have not.

When you first start taking a homeopathic remedy you may experience an initial worsening of the symptoms – an 'aggravation reaction'. This should be short-lived and is a sign the medicine is working.

Homeopathy is also available on the NHS, and your GP can refer you to any of the homeopathic hospitals or to some other approved clinic. He or she can also prescribe homeopathic products for you although these can often be bought more cheaply over the counter. A wide range is available from pharmacists and health food shops. Olivia Hanscombe, who has lupus and, in addition to her extensive personal experience of many complementary therapies, a doctorate in Biochemistry, suggests the following for arthritis:

★ Arnica – for pain in a single joint and gout
★ Rhus-Tox – for rheumatic pains which worsen on rest and ease with gentle movement

For further information contact The Society of Homeopaths (for non-medical homeopaths) or the British Homeopathic Association (for medical homeopaths).

Consumer's report
'I found a local homeopath who had also been a practising doctor. He has started to treat me and generally my condition has

improved overall. He works on the principle of treating the whole person, which I have responded to. My bowel condition is taking a while to improve, but longer-term conditions are known to take longer to sort out. The treatment has given me more energy, a better mental attitude and helped my arthritis slightly. I would say that homeopathy does seem to work for me, but it can take time.'

MASSAGE AND AROMATHERAPY

We all know the benefits of massage. When a child falls over, mummy offers to rub it better. You do the same thing if you have a sore neck or shoulder, probably stretching at the same time. It helps because it can unknot tight muscles, get the body's natural pain-killing endorphins flowing, and block pain messages to the brain. It also helps because it feels good. The human touch is comforting.

The British – some might say the English – are a bit funny about massage. We are not very keen about taking our clothes off in front of strangers at the best of times and anyway, everyone knows that massage parlours are fronts for brothels. Just look at all those adverts for masseuses in the newsagents. Well, forget all that. That's not what therapeutic massage is about.

A gentle massage – the action is a bit like kneading bread – can loosen stiff muscles. A more vigorous, firmer one can tone up slack muscles and stimulate the blood flow. Usually talcum power or a simple oil like coconut is used to help the masseur's hands move smoothly. The Swedish is probably the most widely available technique, but it can, certainly in its traditional and rather structured form, be a little vigorous and possibly painful. A holistic massage, in which the masseur chooses the strokes to suit the individual, is probably more appropriate for people with arthritis.

Aromatherapy is massage with what are called 'essential oils'. These oily extracts are the substance that gives each plant its smell. First used in Pakistan 5,000 years ago, modern

Getting a Grip

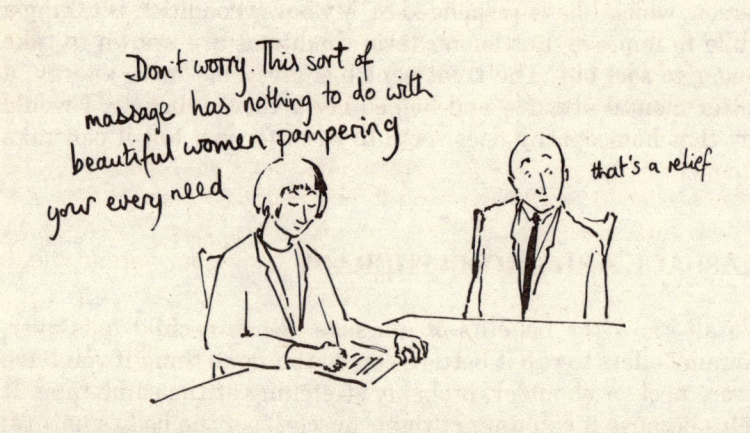

Don't worry. This sort of massage has nothing to do with beautiful women pampering your every need

that's a relief

aromatherapy was developed by a French chemist Rene Maurice Gattefosse. He was working in a perfume factory when he burnt his hand. Panicking, he plunged it into a nearby vat of lavender oil. It healed rapidly and he was left without a scar.

The use of essential oils makes for a more beneficial massage with longer-lasting effects. Each has its own properties – some invigorate, some relax, some reduce inflammation. The skin absorbs them directly. To say nothing of the nose!

There are certain conditions in which a massage may be inappropriate, such as infectious skin complaints, certain spinal injuries and on varicose veins, new scar tissue or the abdomen when pregnant. A good masseur will check on these with you before starting. This is an opportunity to mention the type of massage you'd like – invigorating or relaxing – which areas of the body you'd like particular attention paid to, and which you'd prefer avoided.

The masseur will leave the room while you undress – usually to your underpants. During the massage the body is usually covered with the towels which are removed and replaced as each part of the body is worked on. Tell the masseur immediately if something hurts.

A full body massage lasts up to one and a half hours and costs £25–30. You will usually be left to relax for a moment or two afterwards – perhaps with a glass of water and some music. An aromatherapist will probably ask more questions than a masseur before commencing the treatment. This is to make sure that the appropriate oils are chosen. Two or three are then added to a base oil and used in the massage – which is a gentle one. These oils are quite expensive, so be prepared to pay about £5 more than for a regular massage.

You don't have to have the whole body done – try a hands, feet or face massage.

Massage and aromatherapy have umpteen bodies offering different qualifications, which can be a minefield. To be on the safe side get the list of qualified practitioners from the Institute of Complementary Medicine.

Massage is also something that you can do at home with a friend. For base oils try grape seed (cheap), coconut oil (smells lovely) or sweet almond. If you want essential oils, lavender is the best all-rounder. Rosemary, camomile, juniper and marjoram are also reputed to be good for aches and pains. These are available ready-diluted or mixed in base oils, but it is cheaper if you buy them neat and do it yourself. Dilute three to six drops of essential oil with 10ml of base oil. Be gentle with each other.

You can try acupressure massage, which involves stimulating the acupoints used in acupuncture. This can help blood flow and relaxation.

Remember, stop a massage if it hurts and don't start one on an inflamed joint.

Consumer's report
'Sometimes I like the massage to be quite vigorous as, although this can be initially painful, the relief after a few minutes is indescribable. Deep-seated muscle tension starts to melt away. Joints loosen as muscles let go and relax out of bad positions. My whole body begins to feel pleasantly warm and a sense of peace drifts over my thoughts as the delicate aroma of lavender oil permeates my skin. The effects of a "full-body" last up to a month.'

OSTEOPATHY

Osteopathy is closely related to chiropractic – the founder of the latter training with the founder of the former. Andrew Taylor Still became interested in the mechanics of the body in the 1870s, believing as a Christian that, if man was made in God's image, any problems with the human body must arise from misuse. He also believed that if the correct readjustments were made, the body could heal itself.

Treatment takes place on a low couch. Although osteopathy sees the spine and the joints around it as central to the functioning of the body, most of the treatment will focus on soft tissue, that is the skin, muscle and connective tissue. Contrary to popular perception therefore, it is not unpleasant. Vigorous manipulation resulting in the bones clicking back into position is used sparingly – perhaps once a session.

For people with arthritis, osteopathy is most useful for back and joint pain, particularly with specific joint pain such as a frozen shoulder or at the site of a sports injury. It is also helpful for sciatica.

As with other complementary therapies, osteopathy takes a 'whole-person' approach and practitioners may suggest exercises and different ways of doing things at home and work. On the other hand they don't claim to be able to treat everything. Osteopaths work with bones and muscles and are wary about making broader claims.

At your first appointment, the osteopath, like the chiropractor, will want details of your medical history and your day-to-day life. You will then be examined in a variety of positions: sitting, standing and lying. This initial assessment will take about half an hour and follow-up visits about twenty minutes to half an hour. Sessions cost £15–20.

Finding an osteopath is relatively easy. Most doctors are happy to refer you. In the last year osteopathy has become a regulated profession just like nursing or medicine. For further information contact The General Council and Register of Osteopaths.

Osteopathy is not, of course, a DIY therapy. It should also be avoided if you have osteoporosis, inflamed joints or are in the first three months of pregnancy.

Consumer's report
'Some areas are stretched gently, others manipulated with more force. When a "click" is about to happen, I am asked to breathe in, then out, at which point I am meant to be relaxed. However, this is easier said than done and, although I know the secret is to relax as much as possible, I always find myself tensing in anticipation.

'On the whole, the treatment is uncomfortable rather than painful. After about a week, I start to notice the benefits: my spine is usually straighter and my muscles ache less. I find the effects last for several weeks, although by the time of my next appointment, I am usually ready for treatment.'

REFLEXOLOGY

To the reflexologist, the foot is at the bottom of the problem. Reflexology is a foot massage therapy which has much in common with acupuncture. Sometimes the hands are massaged too.

Each part of the foot corresponds to another part of the body. A reflexologist's plan of the sole of the foot looks like a treasure map. By massaging the appropriate spot the practitioner can stimulate the problematic organ or other part of the body.

Reflexology divides the body into ten reflex zones which run vertically the length of the body. Five are accessed through one foot and five through the other. There are also three horizontal zones. Normally energy flows happily from zone to zone. Problems occur when this flow is blocked. If the reflex zone is healthy, all you will feel when the reflexologist touches the zone on your foot is a little gentle pressure. If it is unhealthy you may feel pain or a mild stabbing sensation. This does not necessarily indicate disease – the problem may be trivial or passing: a little eye strain from watching too much TV before your appointment, for example.

At your first visit, the reflexologist will take a full medical history before the preliminary examination of your feet. You lie on a treatment couch and will obviously need to remove your shoes and socks. Don't worry, it isn't ticklish, even for the most sensitive sole. This first visit lasts about an hour and costs £20 or so. Subsequent sessions last about forty-five minutes and cost £15–20. A treatment once a week for six weeks is usually suggested, with the occasional top-up.

Treatment is very relaxing but you may be surprised to find yourself sweating or feeling shivery. If you feel shivery tell your therapist as this is a sign of over-stimulation. After starting reflexology you may sweat and go to the lavatory more than usual – a good sign, according to reflexologists, that your elimination system is getting into gear. Indeed, the treatment is considered particularly good for bowel and bladder problems.

People with arthritis may also find it useful for improving mobility, easing stress and generally promoting that feel-good factor.

Reflexology is not well regulated. To avoid putting your foot in it, your best bet is the Association of Reflexologists. Their members, who have MAR after their names, must have an approved qualification, a year's experience and a quota of case-histories.

Unless you are an Olympic gymnast, reflexology is hard to practise on yourself. But it's easy to do with a friend. A foot massage from an enthusiastic amateur may not pinpoint your particular problems as a professional might, but it is very relaxing. Press quite firmly and use some talc or oil to make it easier.

Consumer's report
'I found my reflexologist by word of mouth. It was always soothing and gentle. She would ask me about painful joints and sometimes could spot sensitive areas through my feet. I went for about four months, usually once a week or fortnight. It didn't directly help my arthritis, but it helped relax me totally and slowed me right down which was good in itself. I feel it's a shame that more people can't try complementary therapies because of the cost.'

YOGA

Yoga is another discipline that has genuinely passed the test of time. It was practised in India 5,000 years ago. The sacred writings of the Hindu religion, the Vedas, which were written at around that time, contain references to yoga.

It is not a therapy as such – no one practises on you – but something that you can do for yourself. It involves working with your body, your mind and your prana (your vital energy).

There are many types of yoga, but the two main ones are the yoga sutras: raja yoga is meditative, concerned with spiritual enlightenment; whereas hatha yoga is physical, concerned with breathing and the body.

The positions used in yoga, called yoga asanas, have emerged over the centuries as ways to unlock tension, ease stiffness and strengthen weaknesses by freeing the spine and restoring its balance. They move the body in a variety of ways and, along with the correct breathing (called pranayama), stimulate joints and muscles, blood flow, important glands and the digestive and nervous systems.

You no longer need a guru or teacher to practise yoga. Classes are commonly held at leisure centres and evening classes and there are plenty of books available.

For people with arthritis, it can certainly help with relaxation – many people talk of a sense of peace and reduced stress – and may ease stiffness, relax muscles, improve breathing and make you more supple. However, although you can obviously practise at home, it is essential that you discuss it with a professional teacher first. Some positions may not be suitable for your arthritis and you will need to be careful about 'pushing' damaged joints.

There is also much more to yoga for those interested, including teachings on diet, lifestyle, dress and personal habits.

Consumer's report
'Initially I thought yoga may be something I couldn't manage. It has the image of being something done by very fit people. I found a teacher who was very knowledgeable with a long experience of

teaching yoga. She graded the class into different abilities, making the overall experience more comfortable.

'I went along for six sessions and learned things that I still do, such as breathing and stretching exercises. These are similar in some ways to the "Range of movement" exercises that I do for my arthritis but they are much more focused and concentrated, where you think about the rhythm and breathing involved in what you are doing.'

Tai-chi

Similar to yoga, Tai-chi originated in China and is based on the Taoist belief in the forces of Yin and Yang (see acupuncture). It is theoretically a non-violent martial art concerned with balance, concentration and strength. The 'form', a prescribed sequence of movements, is practised solo; 'pushing hands' in pairs. Pushing hands is what it sounds like and, be careful, some teachers can encourage this to be done rather vigorously.

It is more active than yoga, involving movements rather than positions. The stretches are generally more gentle.

Even more so than with yoga, it is important that you talk to a professional Tai-chi instructor who understands arthritis before embarking on a class.

CHAPTER 7

Arthritis and Diet

Can changing what you eat make a difference to your arthritis? Of all the self-help strategies, diet is probably the most controversial. Some people make incredible claims about it; many doctors are still frankly sceptical. On Arthritis Care's telephone helpline it is consistently one of the most popular topics of conversation.

Stop eating red meat, start eating pink gobstoppers and all will be well. If only it were that simple. Don't be tempted by any single diet that claims it will cure arthritis. There isn't one. Everyone's different and everyone's arthritis is different. One of the few things on which everyone reputable in the field agrees is that none of the ideas discussed here work for all of us.

That's not to say that the role of diet isn't important. If we are what we eat then we might be able to alter what we are by altering what we eat. Any doctor will tell you that it's always a good idea to think about what you eat. When you have arthritis, it's perhaps worth thinking about it a little more.

WHAT IS A HEALTHY DIET?

We seem to be bombarded from all sides with advice – eat this, don't eat that, drink more of the other – and much of it is contradictory. However, there are some basic principles, the cornerstones of a healthy diet. Here's what the Health Education Authority says.

A seven-point guide to healthier eating

★ Eat a variety of food to get the full range of nutrients.
★ Eat plenty of foods rich in starch and fibre.
★ Don't eat too much fat.
★ Don't eat sugary foods too often.
★ Look after the vitamins and minerals in your food.
★ If you drink alcohol, keep within sensible levels.
★ Eat the right amount to be a healthy weight.

That's fine, but what is 'too much' or 'too often'? And isn't starch something they put in washing powder? How do you 'look after' vitamins? (Take them for walks?) What is a 'healthy' weight? Let's look at a healthy diet a little more closely.

Fibre and starch

Foods high in fibre and starch should form the main part of most meals. These foods include: bread and rolls; breakfast cereals and oats; pasta and noodles; rice; potatoes and sweet potatoes; dishes made from maize, millet and cornmeal; and beans, pulses and lentils.

Contrary to what you may have heard, these foods are not, of themselves, fattening – although they are filling. The key is how they are cooked. Chips, because they are cooked in fat, contain three times the calories of the same weight of boiled potatoes.

The wholegrain varieties of these starchy foods are a particularly good choice: wholemeal bread, brown rice, wholewheat pasta. They contain more fibre and also more vitamins. Fruit and vegetables also contain fibre, though of a different type – this sort of fibre may help keep down blood cholesterol levels. Try to eat about five portions a day, including some veg, some fruit and some salad.

Include a good mix of all these high-fibre foods in your diet and supplement it with plenty of fluids – aim for at least six to eight drinks daily.

If you are looking to increase the amount of fibre in your diet, try replacing some meat with beans, peas or lentils. Tinned beans of all types will do fine and are more convenient than the dried variety. If you do use dried beans make sure you cook them properly. Kidney beans, for example, need to be soaked for at least five hours! Baked beans are a quick, easy source of fibre.

Fat

While most of us don't eat enough fibre, we generally eat too much fat. A small amount is necessary, but too much may increase the chance of heart disease and obesity.

There are two main types of fat, saturated and unsaturated. It is the saturates that are in the dock over heart disease because they increase the levels of blood cholesterol. Unsaturates are necessary, but in small quantities. Most food contains both types in various quantities. Look for food in which the fat content is low and predominantly unsaturated rather than saturated. Food labels should tell you this.

A third type of fat are trans-fats. These appear to be formed by the hydrogenation process used to turn oils into something spreadable. They may also increase cholesterol, so are best kept to a minimum. If 'hydrogenated vegetable fat/oil' appears on an ingredients list, it means saturates and trans-fats. There are unhydrogenated spreads on the market, although they are not yet widely available.

Foods high in saturated fat include dairy products, meat and fish, hard (and some soft) margarines, cakes, biscuits, chocolates, puddings and savoury snacks.

Foods higher in unsaturated fat include most vegetable oils (sunflower, corn and, particularly, olive and rapeseed), nuts and oily fish (herring, tuna, pilchards, sardines, mackerel and trout).

Fat intake can be reduced by switching to low-fat versions of popular products. Whole milk, for example, contains 22 grams of fat per pint, compared to 0·6 grams in skimmed milk. If you really can't get used to the thinner taste of skimmed, try semi-skimmed (9 grams/pint). All have the same amount of protein and calcium.

The differences can be surprising: fried rice (8 grams of fat in a typical serving) compared to boiled rice (1 gram); pork chop fried (16 grams) or pork chop grilled (6 grams); thin chips of the burger bar variety (17 grams) or baked or boiled potatoes (0.1 gram).

Other possibilities for cutting fat include:

★ switching to a lower-fat margarine (you can compare fat contents by looking at the labels)
★ skipping on spread on bread
★ trying whiter cheeses (they usually have less fat)
★ eating fish and skinless white meat (chicken and turkey) in preference to red meat
★ grilling, microwaving or steaming rather than frying
★ fromage frais instead of cream.

A word about cholesterol
The word is: confusing. Cholesterol is often associated with heart disease, but the relationship is a complicated one. Cholesterol eaten in food does not automatically turn into cholesterol in the blood, and it is this blood cholesterol that can be dangerous.

Because cholesterol is fat and cannot dissolve there are two things that can be done with: it can stay in the body or be excreted. Cholesterol is carried around the blood by special molecules called lipoproteins. The low-density lipoproteins (LDLs) dump their cholesterol on the artery walls. It is these deposits, called plaque, that are implicated in heart disease. However, high-density lipoproteins (HDLs) take their cholesterol to the liver where it can eventually be excreted.

It is more accurate to talk of LDL cholesterol, sometimes called 'bad' cholesterol, and HDL, 'good' cholesterol. It is the former that is stashed away in saturated fats and trans-fats. It is the latter that is boosted by exercise.

Vitamins and minerals
By following the seven-point guide at the start of this section you should get all the vitamins and minerals you need without supplements. These are often expensive and, what's more, although standard doses should not be dangerous, too much of

certain vitamins (particularly A and D) can cause problems.

You can maximise the benefit from the vitamins in your food by keeping it as fresh as possible and storing it carefully. Paper rather than plastic bags are better for fridge storage. There are also special bags, called Evergreen, available for keeping veg fresh.

Frozen, chilled, dried or packaged foods can be just as good a source of vitamins as fresh foods. Again, store properly and follow the directions on the pack.

We lose a lot of the nutrients in vegetables by over-cooking them – cook both fresh and frozen varieties for as short a time in as little water as possible. Or use the microwave.

Alcohol

Certain drugs may prevent you from drinking anyway, but if you are able to, watch your units. One unit of alcohol equals a half-pint of regular beer or a small sherry or a glass of wine or a single measure of spirits. Men should not exceed twenty-one units a week, while women, rather unfairly, should draw the line at fourteen. Alcohol is very high in calories – a pint of beer contains about 180, a glass of wine, ninety-five.

Sugar and salt

You should get enough of these from your regular diet. Sugar contains nothing but calories – albeit very nice ones – and will damage your teeth. Cutting sugar is the easiest way to cut calories without losing nutrients.

Most of us should reduce our salt intake by about a third – use less in cooking, don't automatically salt your food, and choose tinned vegetables with 'no added salt'.

Weight

If you are able to do all these things, you should wind up the right weight for your height. This is particularly important for people with arthritis. Keeping your weight down, particularly if you have osteoarthritis, will really help. For example, every pound you put on round your tummy adds an extra four pounds to the weight put through your knee every time you take a step.

There is evidence to suggest that your chances of developing osteoarthritis can be as much as halved by being within 10% of your ideal body weight. Clearly, being the correct weight also brings benefits if you already have the disease.

If you are overweight, the risks of heart disease, high blood pressure and diabetes are greater. To lose weight, cut calories without cutting nutrients.

★ Eat filling, lower-calorie foods – that is, those higher in fibre.
★ Cut fat – it has twice as many calories gram for gram as protein or starch.
★ Stop using sugar.
★ Avoid sweetened drinks, sugary, fatty foods and alcohol.
★ Burn off more calories – that is, take more exercise.

If you are underweight, you may not be getting all the nutrients necessary for good health.

Height–Weight Chart
How close are you to your ideal weight? Weigh yourself without clothes and shoes. Measure yourself without shoes. If you are more than a stone (14lb) overweight you will, in the words of Dr Vernon Coleman, 'almost certainly be having an adverse effect on your joints'. In truth, you probably will even if you are less overweight than that.

Ideal weight range for women

HEIGHT	WEIGHT
4' 10"	7st. 5lbs – 8st. 5lbs
5' 0"	7st. 9lbs – 8st. 9lbs
5' 2"	8st. 1lb – 9st. 1lb
5' 4"	8st. 6lbs – 9st. 6lbs
5' 6"	9st. 0lbs – 10st. 0lbs
5' 8"	9st. 7lbs – 10st. 7lbs
5' 10"	10st. 0lbs – 11st. 0lbs
6' 0"	10st. 7lbs – 11st. 7lbs

Ideal weight range for men

HEIGHT	WEIGHT
5' 0"	8st. 5lbs – 9st. 5lbs
5' 2"	8st. 7lbs – 9st. 7lbs
5' 4"	8st. 11lbs – 9st. 11lbs
5' 6"	9st. 6lbs – 10st. 6lbs
5' 8"	10st. 0lbs – 11st. 0lbs
5' 10"	10st. 8lbs – 11st. 8lbs
6' 0"	11st. 2lbs – 12st. 2lbs
6' 2"	11st. 10lbs – 12st. 10lbs
6' 4"	12st. 4lbs – 13st. 4lbs

Food labels

Labels are a vital source of information about what you are eating, but they can be misleading. Many descriptions commonly used on foods have no legal definitions – manufacturers can use them to mean what they want.

Recently, one of the largest hamburger chains revealed that by the word 'nutritious', they didn't mean necessarily that the food was good for you, only that it contained 'nutrients'. Big deal. Virtually all food, even the unhealthiest imaginable, contains some nutrients. It's the same with 'low fat' and 'high fibre'. They could mean anything. The European Community is looking to regulate this, but it hasn't happened yet. At present, by law all that has to be included is weight, a list of ingredients in weight order and cooking and storage instructions.

More useful is the nutritional information given on packets. It usually provides the amount of each nutrient in the whole product and per 100 grams. This enables you to compare one food with another.

★ Energy – the number of calories in the product.

★ Carbohydrate – starches and sugar. More helpful labels will say 'of which sugars' which will tell you how much of the carbohydrate total is sugar. The rest will be starch. Go for low sugar.

★ Fat – again, a helpful label should give a separate figure for *'contains harmless edible nutrients with extra vitamins and added fibre'...*

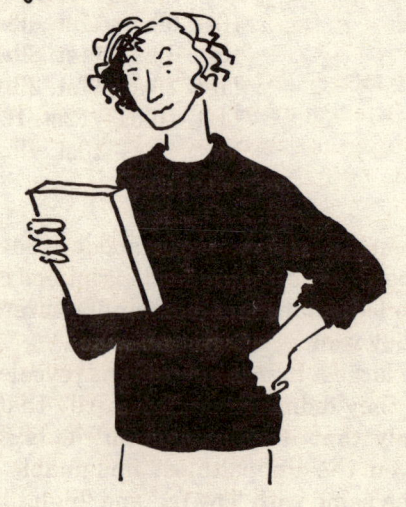

saturates. The rest should be unsaturates. Go for the lowest amount of saturates.
★ Sodium – broadly, how much salt. Go for low sodium products.
★ The labels should also tell you how much fibre and protein is in the product. Go for high fibre, high protein.

For more information on a healthy diet, ask your GP or local health education authority.

The biggest single thing that most people can do in terms of diet is to make sure it's a balanced and healthy one. While this may need to be modified for some people with arthritis, all the ideas in the rest of this chapter take a healthy basic diet as their starting point.

DIET AND ARTHRITIS

There are two areas worth thinking about here:

★ dietary supplements
★ dietary manipulation

It is important to stress that real scientific research is still in its infancy in this area. Relatively little has been done – most of it on rheumatoid arthritis. The leading rheumatologist working in this field is Dr Gail Darlington, who gives her verdict on each supplement at the end.

Diet supplements and rheumatoid arthritis

★ **Fish oils** – The fatty acids in fish oil may produce less inflammatory chemicals than those from animal fats, suggesting that fish oil may thereby ease joint pain and stiffness. It takes three to six months to become effective and needs to be taken long-term. Cod-liver oil is taken by many people with arthritis and the tablets are considerably more palatable than the liquid some readers may remember enduring as children!

However, long-term safety has yet to be investigated. As has the effect of the lower-strength doses that you can buy over the counter. (The major controlled test was on high doses of cod-liver oil.) What can be said with more certainty is that fish oil is good for your heart. Fish oils are not available on prescription and can be expensive.

Dr Darlington's verdict: 'Promising'.

★ **Evening Primrose Oil (EPO)** – Evening Primrose Oil is extracted from the Evening Primrose, a beautiful little yellow flower that only comes out at night! EPO has similar effects to fish oil and also takes from three to six months to become effective. Similarly, long-term effects have yet to be investigated. Fish oils and EPO can be taken together. It seems that both help the production of anti-inflammatory prostaglandins in the body although by different paths.

Dr Darlington's verdict: 'Promising'.

★ **New Zealand green-lipped Mussel** – This product may have a mild anti-inflammatory effect, although evidence of its value in RA is limited.

Dr Darlington's verdict: 'No certain evidence'.

★ **Selenium** – There is some evidence of a relationship between low levels of the trace element selenium and arthritis, but its nature is unclear and appears not to be straightforward. Selenium by mouth may be toxic in large quantities – as may any mineral.

Dr Darlington's verdict: 'Uncertain value by mouth'.

★ **Iron** – Anaemia in RA does not necessarily respond to iron supplements.

Dr Darlington's verdict: 'Discuss with your doctor'.

★ **Garlic** – Fresh garlic (rather than pearls) is good for the heart, if not for your personal relationships, but its benefit in RA is not yet known.

Dr Darlington's verdict: 'Insufficient serious studies'.

Dietary manipulation in RA
Dietary manipulation will only work for some people with rheumatoid arthritis (Dr Darlington puts the figure at about 40% of people with RA). It takes about six weeks and involves removing from your diet certain foods which contribute to your symptoms.

If you try this it must be under medical supervision from a doctor or medical homeopath, because there is a danger of malnutrition. It can also be disruptive to your life and needs a high level of commitment. If it doesn't work after six weeks it is important to return to your existing treatment to avoid joint damage. There are three stages:

★ Elimination – removing from your diet all foods which might be causing symptoms – this tends to mean pretty much all foods, which is why medical supervision is so important.
★ Reintroduction – if symptoms do disappear, foods are reintroduced to see if they cause the symptoms to return.
★ Challenging – once the probable culprits have been discovered, challenging involves checking out by removal and reintroduction if they really are the cause of the symptoms. To avoid a placebo response, this is best done without your knowledge (although this is difficult with some types of food!). This third phase is particularly important because initial benefits may simply be the result of the natural ups and downs of rheumatoid arthritis or a placebo response, or it may be your body responding to its initial starvation by increasing its own production of corticosteroids.

Barry Hayward used diet to help control rheumatoid arthritis for eight years. 'I was fed up with taking drugs. I was on Prednisolene. It wasn't that they weren't working but I'd been on drugs for eight years. It was also a hassle having to carry them everywhere with you all the time – you couldn't be spontaneous.

'I met a woman who had been to a food allergy clinic and she found it so good I decided to give it a try. I was getting into healthier eating anyway. It was run by Dr John Mansfield [author of *Arthritis: The Allergy Connection*]. For the first week to ten days, they put you on a very simple, preferably uncooked, vegetable diet – I remember carrots, grapes and pears. They said that initially you should feel worse as your system clears and then you'll notice an improvement. What appealed to me about it was that they said if you don't have this dip then it probably isn't going to work for you. That meant I had nothing much to lose – I'd know fairly quickly whether it was worth pursuing.

'It did work. I felt much better. When I began to reintroduce another food, I could tell within a couple of hours if it was affecting me. It's not like those therapies where you can't really tell if it's working. With this you really can.

'I also did skin tests which are used for more complicated allergies such as monosodium glutamate and yeast – the things you cannot test so easily by mouth. The tests are expensive though. Avoiding additives, sugar and wheat worked for me – when I felt bad I could usually trace it to one of these.

'Something else they suggest is taking a very tiny diluted dose of the food to which you are allergic to suppress the allergy temporarily – similar to homeopathy. I was more sceptical about this and it didn't work for me with bread. I'm in remission now so I've stopped watching my diet in the same way but it was certainly very helpful for me at the time.'

Hilary Walters, who has a less precisely diagnosed form of inflammatory arthritis, agrees. 'I went to the Glasgow Homeopathic Hospital about four years ago and an exclusion diet was suggested. I was keen to try non-drug, whole person type therapies.

'We talked about personality – foods you like, foods you don't like. I excluded all meat, all wheat, all sugar, potatoes, tomatoes, green peppers, all citrus fruits and shellfish for several weeks. I didn't really notice any difference at this stage. I think these things had been in my system so long. I then started reintroducing food groups for a week at a time – if there was no reaction you could carry on eating them.

'They suggested that you reintroduce the foods you eat a lot of first as these are often the ones you are sensitive to. I introduced dairy produce but it wasn't that. In fact, wheat was about the last one I reintroduced and I realised within an hour that that was what it was. I was totally exhausted – it was like flu. But at last I'd found something I could do. I was in more control. I think the initial cleansing out of your system is emotionally beneficial too.

'I stuck to a no-wheat diet rigidly for about two years and now I can get away with the odd bit of sinning – an occasional biscuit or cake.'

Diet and osteoarthritis

As we have said, there is a relationship between arthritis and weight, so a diet that keeps you at your ideal weight for your height can help. Talk to your GP for advice on losing weight. You might want to think about joining a slimming group.

Diet and ankylosing spondylitis

Research is being undertaken into a variety of diets for people with ankylosing spondylitis, but nothing certain has yet emerged.

Diet and systemic lupus erythematosus

A low-fat, high-fish-oil diet may help some people with SLE.

Diet and osteoporosis

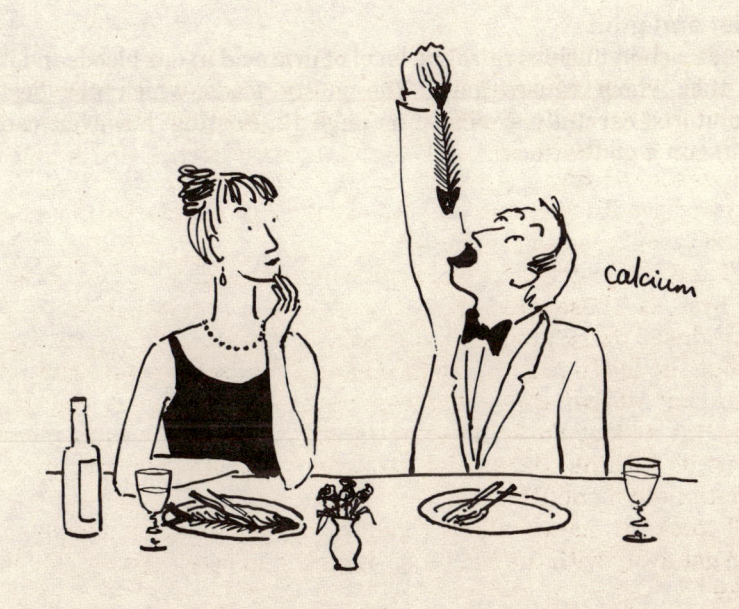

Calcium and vitamin D are essential for strong, healthy bones. Although this need is greatest in childhood, you can still help to protect against osteoporosis as an adult. Calcium tablets may be useful, but you need to check with your doctor that your tablets provide it in sufficient quantities. Take plenty of liquid with your tablet.

Most adults need about 800mg of calcium a day. However, younger adults, expectant or recent mothers, women after the menopause and men over sixty-five may require more: up to 1500mg. The usual sources of calcium are dairy products.

★ A 235ml cup of milk (either skimmed, semi-skimmed or full cream) contains about 300mg of calcium.
★ A 235ml cup of low-fat yogurt contains about 400mg of calcium.
★ One ounce of cheddar cheese contains about 200mg of calcium.

Other foods rich in calcium include broccoli, tofu, some types of beans, almonds and canned fish including mackerel, salmon and sardines (if eaten with the bones in).

Diet and gout
Foods rich in purines raise the level of uric acid in our blood, and it is this which causes gout. The guilty foods which are best monitored carefully are listed on page 12. Fasting, however, can bring on a gout attack.

CHAPTER 8

Arthritis and the Mind

'It's all in the mind' – how often have you heard that expression? It may have been applied to you. It's an easy way to dismiss something we don't understand.

Perhaps sometimes even you think your arthritis is all in the mind – when you're having a good day. Arthritis is an up and down affair and often its effects are invisible. You can never see pain; you can't always see joint damage. One day you can hardly move, the next you're strolling off to the shops and, apart from the smile on your face, you don't look any different. No wonder we all get a little sceptical sometimes about just how serious arthritis is.

If you're keeping a journal of your drugs and doctor's appointments, here's another use for it: recording how you feel. You could use a pain scale like that mentioned on page 48.

Have you ever felt yourself thinking, 'There are plenty of people worse than me'? Sometimes we belittle or trivialise how we feel in a misplaced display of altruism. I say misplaced because this attitude is not actually doing anything for those people who are 'worse' than you anyway. It's simply an excuse not to do anything about your own disease. Sure there probably are people who are 'worse' (whatever that means) than you, but if you really want to help them, all the more reason to make sure you are managing your own arthritis as well as you can.

What about the athlete who quits because 'there are plenty of people better than me'? Or the musician? It's just an excuse for not trying, and 'there are plenty of people worse than me' is just the same.

The fact is that whatever you do, you're only going to succeed if you give it your best shot. It is as true with arthritis as it is with athletics. If you want to exercise more control over your arthritis, however mild or severe it is, you will only do it if you take it seriously. And, like the athlete, like the musician, it helps if you are able to practise every day.

'But I'm not really disabled.' Okay, but so what? What do you mean by 'disabled' anyway? Our general perception, created and reinforced by the media and to some extent the medical profession, is that disability is a terrible state. Many people when they are first diagnosed as having arthritis are worried that they will 'end up in a wheelchair'. They won't – only a small minority of people with arthritis use wheelchairs. But hidden in the fear is the belief that severe disability is the worse thing that can happen to you – a belief encouraged by media stories of 'triumph over tragedy' or 'children of courage'. A friend said, 'When I got arthritis, my mother thought the world had come to an end.'

In fact, many severely disabled people are very positive about their experience. They feel it has given them new skills, developed their characters and given them a greater understanding and insight into themselves and others.

Traditionally, 'disabled' is seen as the opposite of 'able-bodied' or 'coping normally'. It is more helpful and accurate to see it as different. Many disabled people cope with life far more successfully than many 'normal' people. Don't run scared of the disabled label. Being disabled does not mean being a burden, not being normal, or not coping. Indeed, the psychological problems involved in fighting it may cause more problems than any associated with embracing it.

Of course, none of this by itself will change other people's views of disability – but these are based in ignorance and fear, not in fact. On the other hand, ignorance can only be overcome if it is challenged.

Two definitions:

★ Impairment – a body part or function that doesn't work properly or is missing.

★ Disability – the resulting lack of function.

Because you are impaired by arthritis, you may as a result be unable to use stairs. A ramp or a lift or even a grab-rail may be able to reduce or remove your disability. It is therefore much more helpful and accurate to see disability as a social phenomenon rather than a personal thing. If you say 'I am disabled' you are in many important respects making more of a statement about the society in which we live than about yourself.

There are many occasions when acknowledging the disability you have is beneficial. Gadgets 'for disabled people' can lessen that disability. Registering or being eligible to register as a 'disabled person' can help with work and Social Services. More on these in Chapter 11.

It's no wonder we tend to shy away from the word 'disabled', given the negative overtones that we tend to put on it. The words used to describe us, whether by ourselves or others, play a big part in how we feel about ourselves. It's understandable that we don't want to feel negative about ourselves. The negative associations with the word 'disabled' are artificial or inaccurate, but that is not always the case.

If you use negative terms to describe yourself or allow others to apply them to you, you could well start feeling negative about yourself. Many people with arthritis feel like this about 'sufferer', for example. Sufferers are passive, people to whom unpleasant things happen. Is that how you see yourself? Or want others to? Many people feel the same about describing themselves as a medical condition – the word 'arthritic' allows the disease to swamp the person. That is why most people simply call themselves people with arthritis. Because they are people first – not victims and not medical conditions.

These concerns about the words we use have nothing to do with what the newspapers call 'political correctness' and everything to do with developing a positive self-image.

SELF-IMAGE

How we feel about ourselves has a big impact on how others feel about us and on how far we feel able to do the things that we want to do. We all benefit from a positive self-image. That's true for everybody. But it's hard and, when you have arthritis, it can be doubly so.

It's a vicious circle. How we feel about ourselves affects how we present ourselves. How we present ourselves affects how others see us. How others see us affects how we feel about ourselves.

If others see people with disabilities such as arthritis as somehow second rate, as victims, as incomplete or as not whole, that is going to have an impact on your self-esteem. These views are encouraged and reinforced in the media. Not just in the way they present 'disability' as a tragedy to be triumphed over but in their whole value system: the real man fixes his car – not easy when you have arthritis; the proper woman comforts her baby – fine so long as the baby's not too heavy; and both must aspire to the ad-man's dream of perfect skin and bones – well, it's just not possible is it?

No wonder self-image takes a battering. To break the vicious circle, it's necessary to go back to the start. You can't control what others think about you, but you can control what you think about yourself.

A positive self-image is the foundation for managing your arthritis and there's nothing wrong with involving other people in your search for it. Counselling or self-help groups in which you can meet with other people with arthritis can both help. Both are discussed later in this chapter. There is more on self-esteem in Chapter 10.

Positive thinking books may be useful too, although you need to find a style that suits you. Some can be absurdly individualistic in their approach, suggesting that your arthritis is a result of your own negativity and that by adopting the right mental approach (i.e. the one in the book) you will be able to secure world peace, cure the common cold, score a hat-trick for Manchester United and still be home in time to cook the perfect meal for your six children and indolent husband.

There is an excellent discussion of all the issues around self-image in the Young Arthritis Care booklet *Our Relationships, Our Sexuality* by Kata Kolbert.

YOUR ARTHRITIS IS YOUR BUSINESS

Taking steps to exercise more control over your arthritis is often called 'self-help' or 'self-management'. The self-management concept is a useful one. To understand it, think about management in its more general sense – of a business, say. What does a manager do? These are some of the tasks carried out by a manager of any business – you may well be able to think of more.

★ Set goals based on the company's objectives.
★ Determine what needs to be done to meet those goals.
★ Make short-term and long-term plans based on these strategies.
★ Check on progress of the plans.
★ Change them as necessary.

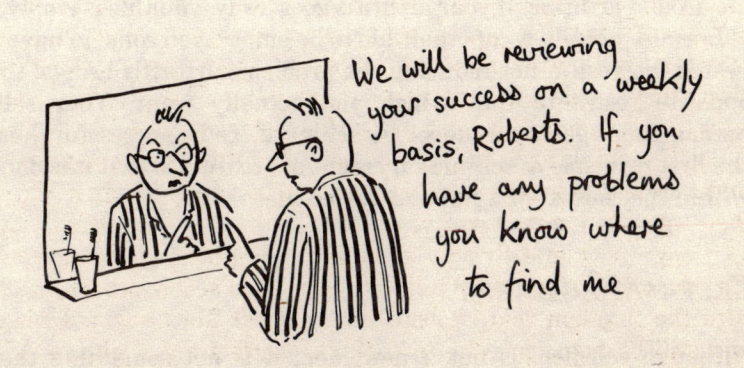

Your arthritis is your business and you can do the same. That's all very well, but how do you make it happen? If a business manager fails to do these things, the business goes bust. If you fail, your life will carry on. In the end, of course, it's a question of will-power, a question of wanting it (think of the athlete again).

Another idea from the business world can make it easier. Just as a business makes contracts with its employees, make contracts with yourself. A contract can include what you are going to do, how often you are going to do it, and when and where. A contract can cover any aspect of your life that you want it to: diet, exercise, complementary therapies, meditation, sex . . .

Like any good contract, it should include some return or reward.

The other side of the coin

There is another side to the arthritis coin. Take it seriously, but don't build your life around it. You are a person, not a business.

Let me give a personal example of what I mean. When I was worried about going freelance, a friend recommended to me a book. It had a very appropriate title for my situation: *Feel the Fear and Do It Anyway*. It's about taking power in your life – much as we've been talking about here – and, at one point, the author Susan Jeffers writes about how to make your life fuller.

She gives the example of people who build their whole lives around a relationship – a marriage or a love affair. When the relationship ends, life is empty. To avoid this overdependency on one aspect of your life, Jeffers urges dividing your life up into interrelated segments. Similarly, think about what happens when you build your life around arthritis. If your arthritis goes away, your life is empty.

Because nobody wants their life to be empty, you come to have a vested interest in not reducing the problems arthritis brings: the opposite result to that which you actually want. Your self-management goals can never be achieved. To be successful then, the first principle of self-management of arthritis is that it is done within the context of a full and varied life.

SELF-MANAGEMENT

Although self-help is not a new idea, it is not something that doctors, until recently, have particularly encouraged for people with arthritis. There are probably two reasons for this.

The first is the non-holistic approach of western medicine. Unlike many of the complementary therapies discussed in Chapter 6 which are holistic (that is to say they believe that it is necessary to treat the whole person in order to ease a particular problem), traditional medicine in this country treats symptoms. The growth in popularity and the success of some complementary therapies has resulted in more and more people, doctors and patients alike, recognising the importance of a 'whole person', body and mind, approach. Self-help is a key part of this.

The second reason is that the understandable obsession of researchers with finding a cure for the various diseases such as arthritis has left people who already have the diseases in second place.

This is particularly true in the case of arthritis. The Arthritis and Rheumatism Council (ARC) spends millions every year (£16 million in 1994) on research – and progress is slow. In the process, ARC produce some very useful patient-education material but they are primarily a research organisation. A registered charity, ARC is twenty-fourth in the league table which ranks charities by their fund-raising capacity. In football terms, the ARC is just about in the premiership. Ironically, much of that money for research is attracted by exploiting the public's fears: using just the sort of images of pity and tragedy that can be so damaging to the self-image of those who actually have the disease. It's for this reason that people with arthritis, and many other disabilities, are demanding more of a say in the organisations that purport to exist for their benefit.

Equally dependent on donations is Arthritis Care, a voluntary organisation committed to working with the eight million Britons who already have arthritis. It's seventy-third in the fund-raising league – division two. The positions of these two voluntary organisations reflects the traditional primacy of research over welfare.

Things are changing. Decades of campaigning by minority groups of all types means that central and local government policy is now far more people-centred. Consultation with users, for example, is built into the Community Care system introduced by the Government in 1993. Arthritis Care itself has recently conducted widespread research into meeting the needs of all people with arthritis. It now offers a whole range of self-help and self-management courses for people with arthritis of all ages and from all sections of the community.

In the USA, where they've always been much better at asking for what they want than we have, such courses are well established. Arthritis Care's are based on those developed at Stanford University by Kate Lorig and attended by thousands of Americans with arthritis. The courses are recommended by the American organisations, the Arthritis Foundation and the Arthritis Society. Kate came over to the UK for the initial training of the Arthritis Care trainers. Her excellent book, *The Arthritis Helpbook*, written with James Fries, has been invaluable in writing this book and is mentioned in the selected reading list in Chapter 13.

The three principles of Kate Lorig's Arthritis Self-help classes are:

★ Everyone with arthritis is different. There is no one treatment that is right for everyone.
★ There are a number of things people can do to feel better. These things will not cure most kinds of arthritis, but they will help to relieve pain, maintain or increase mobility, and prevent deformity.
★ With knowledge, each individual is the best judge of which self-management techniques are best for him or her.

PAIN

While self-image may be affected by others, pain really is something that is all in the mind. Now, don't get me wrong; I'm not minimising pain. In Arthritis Care's membership survey, 97% of people said they had experienced pain in the previous week. But it is a fact: it's all in the mind.

Pain messages, along with all the other sensations we may feel, travel down nerve fibres to the spinal cord which acts as a sort of information superhighway straight to the brain. Not surprisingly, there's quite a bit of congestion around the spinal cord and, as with any highway, there's a limit to the number of messages that can complete their journey to the central nervous system in the brain at any one time. This congestion, unlike that at the end of your road, can be used to your advantage.

In the 1960s, scientists Ronald Melzack and Patrick Wall put forward the 'gate theory of pain'. They suggested that non-pain sensations travel along thicker nerve fibres than pain sensations, and that they travel more quickly. Because not every message to the brain can get through the 'gate' at the same time it is possible, by bombarding the gate with non-pain messages, to stop the painful ones getting through.

This may all sound like science fiction, but it does explain a lot of things with which we are all familiar – why so many people seriously injured (in accidents, for example) do not, at first, feel pain, and why rubbing a painful spot helps ease it.

But pain has had a bad press. It's important not to lose sight of its purpose. Pain tells you that something is wrong – it tells you you have burned yourself, cut yourself, broken your leg and so on.

After exercise, it can let you know when you've pushed it too far. In your joints, it signals inflammation and possible damage. In your stomach, it can be an early warning of gastric problems. It can be dangerous to ignore pain. That said, we all know it can also be very, very unpleasant to live with continually. In the Arthritis Care members survey, 37% said they were in constant pain. This can be mentally damaging too, leading to depression, anxiety and insecurity. So, how can you close the pain gate?

Closing the pain gate

Drugs: Some drugs, such as aspirin and paracetamol, work by preventing the pain sensations from ever setting off on their journey to the central nervous system. Others, the narcotic analgesics such as codeine, work by allowing the pain signals through the gate but then kidding the brain that they are something else. Drugs are covered in detail in Chapter 5.

Rubbing it better: This works because the rubbing sensation beats the pain sensation to the gate. The more sophisticated applications of this technique to relieve arthritis through massage, shiatsu or the TENS machine are covered in Chapter 6.

Occupying the mind: Keeping the mind busy prevents the pain messages swarming around unhindered. That's why as full a life as possible really does help arthritis. Doing something interesting can, of course, occupy the mind, but you need to balance activity with relaxation. When relaxing it is equally important to keep the mind focused on what you want it to focus on. Think about anything you like, providing you enjoy it. It could be what you'll be doing in the future or something you have done in the past. It may be your family and friends or your hobbies. Use your imagination. For more focused uses of the mind in relaxation and meditation, see below.

Heat: We all know how relaxing a long hot bath can be. The 'warmth' messages, like the 'rubbing' message when you rub a joint better, beat the pain messages to the gate. Heat also stimulates the blood flow. As well as bathing, you could try:
★ electric blankets
★ thicker sheets, flannelette, for example
★ a hot towel, or a hot water bottle wrapped in a towel
★ a sun lamp
★ heating clothes on a radiator before putting them on
★ heated pads – pads are available for various parts of the body. Some run off the mains, others use batteries or are heated in the microwave and some are operated with a special disc in the pad itself. Special features include thermostats and a massage facility. Be careful. Some of these products are unscrupulously priced. Also check that anything you buy is approved to BEAB (British) or CCA (European) standards.

★ asking your physiotherapist about diathermy – a safe deep-heat treatment for the joints.

Cold: Curiously, cold also works for some people, particularly during a flare-up of symptoms. It can reduce swelling and muscle spasms. It helps by having a numbing, anaesthetising effect and may encourage the body to produce its own pain-killing endorphins. Cold packs are available at the pharmacist's, or you can make your own by wrapping a damp towel around a pack of frozen vegetables or a bag of crushed ice. Or you could try an ice-filled hot water bottle! Frozen veg is excellent as you can enjoy them (and all their vitamins and minerals) for your tea afterwards. Keep the ice-pack moving over the skin to prevent ice burns. Stop when it feels numb and don't apply ice directly.

Sleep: A good night's sleep will really help. The problem is that pain is usually at its worst from around ten o'clock, making it difficult to drop off. Altering your sleep patterns might help: going to bed earlier or taking an afternoon nap. Avoid stimulants such as alcohol, cigarettes, tea or coffee in the couple of hours before going to bed. Try a warm bath instead. Make sure that you will be warm, comfortable (most people with arthritis prefer a firmer bed) and will not be disturbed (try ear-plugs if necessary).

Sex: One of the best ways of closing the pain gate and probably the most enjoyable one to try. More about this in Chapter 10.

Pain clinics
There are now over 200 pain clinics across the UK. A directory of these is available from the College of Health, price £10. Many are attached to hospitals. They were set up by anaesthetists and nurses and others to raise awareness of and meet the needs of people with pain – something the NHS has traditionally accorded low priority.

Rosalie Everatt, the director of self-help group Pain-Wise UK, says in Arthritis Care's special magazine *Talk About Pain*, that people with chronic pain 'become known as "thick-file" or "heart-sink" patients as we're parcelled around from specialist to physiotherapist to GP and maybe psychiatrist'. Pain clinics strive to offer a whole-person approach to pain management, including many of the approaches outlined in this book. However, quality is variable and there are no government or professional regulations controlling them at present.

Rebecca Cassidy has experienced the good and the bad. 'I used to attend a pain clinic at the hospital, run by an anaesthetist who was understanding, caring and keen to try different methods of pain control if something didn't work. His support gave me great encouragement.

'When I moved house I was near a pain clinic of world renown. I thought things could only improve. Prior to my appointment I had to complete a lengthy questionnaire. The doctor I saw glanced through what I had written. He poured scorn on my answers, saying that what prevented me from doing something was my will, not my pain. I had always understood the philosophy of pain clinics to be "Pain is what the patient says it is", but this doctor made me feel a complete fraud. He said I must be depressed and that would increase my perception of pain. I said the only reason I felt depressed was because doctors wouldn't listen to me.'

STRESS

Closely related to pain is stress. One can lead to the other. Indeed there appears to be some relationship between very high stress and the onset of rheumatoid arthritis. Like pain, stress also has a purpose. The right amount keeps us mentally alert, motivates us and can boost energy, but too much can be dangerous.

Stress raises the heart-rate, boosting the flow of adrenalin (a natural stimulant) and of cortisone (a painkiller) in the blood system, but also the level of cholesterol. A lot of stress over a long period can produce symptoms of nervousness, headache, sweating, fatigue, faintness, neck and chest pain and breathing difficulties. It can also put the immune system under unnecessary pressure. As with pain, everyone has their own individual stress threshold. Try to develop an armoury of relaxation techniques to cope when you reach yours. You can also try to see stress off at the pass by identifying which activities make you feel stressful and trying to keep them apart from each other: ensuring work and domestic deadlines don't clash, for instance.

Admitting to feeling stressed can be seen as a sign of weakness in our high-speed go-get-it society, but it isn't. Again try to listen honestly to your body.

RELAXATION

Getting the right balance between rest and exercise is difficult but important. Without exercise, muscles become weak and the body flabby, increasing the chances of problems when you do finally move. On the other hand, rest is important for joint protection and pain control. Try to listen to your body honestly and learn to recognise the difference between the need to rest and the desire to be lazy. And don't get hung up on being brave.

Pain and stress can cause the muscles to tighten, affect breathing and increase your pulse and blood pressure. Relaxing can reverse these effects and put you back in control.

There are many techniques you can learn to relax but they do take time. You need to be somewhere you feel comfortable and with some time to yourself. Sit or lie in a comfortable position and close your eyes. Some soothing background music may help (you can buy special relaxation tapes or have a browse in the New Age section of your local music shop). Breathe slowly and deeply, concentrating on your breathing. Think of relaxing words – peace, calm, quiet, contentment – and repeat them to yourself. In meditation, this repetition is called a mantra.

Unconvinced? If it's because you think it sounds silly then you're quite right. But that doesn't mean it doesn't work. Give it a try. If it's because you think it's self-indulgent to take time out just for yourself, think again: any doctor will tell you that a little pampering is good for you. Why not pamper yourself? Strictly for medicinal purposes, of course! If you don't think you'll have enough time, don't worry. Little and often is excellent. Ten minutes a day will do fine.

MEDITATION

Meditation and other more advanced relaxation techniques are very popular with those who have been able to invest the time to master them. Although relaxation has real mental benefits, it focuses primarily on the body; eastern meditation focuses directly on the mind.

Meditation is practised with the spine upright, allowing the body to be alert. It can be learned from a teacher or using a tape or a book. It involves 'detached observation' – seeing everything, judging nothing. For example, look at yourself in the mirror. Concentrate on just looking at yourself, your image, without making any mental comment on it.

Geraldine Anderson, who meditates twice daily for twenty minutes at a time, says: 'When you find thoughts getting in the way, just return to counting your breaths or repeating your mantra. You are still aware of your surroundings but sometimes you will find that you are neither thinking, reciting nor counting. This is what is known as pure consciousness.

'Meditation has often been described as diving into deep water. Gravity draws you down, the technique simply gives you the right angle.'

Practise some of the meditation techniques mentioned below. They've all been tried by people with arthritis who have found them to be restful, refreshing and soothing. It can help put you in control of your emotions rather than the other way round. They all require perseverance.

★ Visualisation – In visualisation (or guided imagery) a voice on a tape may take you on a journey through a beautiful garden or by a seashore or down a country lane, and you are encouraged to imagine yourself in these peaceful surroundings. With practice you may be able to guide yourself.

★ Focused breathing – Focus on the air moving in and out of your nostrils or the rise and fall of your chest. Silently count each breath if you like.

★ Mantra meditation – Repeat a word or phrase that works for you (see Relaxation above).

★ Concentrative meditation – Without blinking, focus on a small object about a metre away. Close your eyes and let your mind picture the object. When it fades begin again.

Meditation and relaxation are of benefit to everyone, but can be particularly useful to people with arthritis. Detached observation can help overcome any negative feelings we have about ourselves. Meditation is a proven pain-controller. In one admittedly rather intensive study, over half of the participants halved their pain scores and three-quarters reduced their drug intake. Most importantly, people who meditate often say that while the pain is still there, their feelings towards it have changed. There are many books on meditation.

COUNSELLING AND PSYCHOTHERAPY

In this country we may say that a problem shared is a problem halved, but we're incredibly reluctant actually to act on it. Talking about our problems, especially to an outsider with the prefix 'psycho-' in his job title, is seen as a sign of failure. It isn't. It isn't giving up or asking someone else to sort your problems out for you. Quite the opposite. It's a way of regaining control of your life.

Counselling is non-judgemental. The counsellor will try to empathise with your problems but won't say 'I think you should do this'. It can help you reclaim your self-respect and put you in a position to make and act upon your own decisions.

Counselling can help with specific problems which are causing stress or unhappiness in your life. Psychotherapy, which has the same person-centred approach but can be more analytical, is probably more appropriate for longer-term problems.

In both cases, the answers will come from you – the client. The counsellor or therapist simply creates a talking environment in which you can do this. Essentially this will involve looking at where you are now, looking at where you want to be, and then looking at how you might get there.

Lida Clark, one of the Arthritis Care's telephone counsellors, says: 'Counselling can be useful for people with arthritis in that it can offer the opportunity to express the anger and frustration that many people can experience. It can also offer a useful opportunity to explore self-management programmes and changes in lifestyle.'

Finding the right counsellor for you is very important. For a list of registered counsellors contact the British Association for Counselling. Be wary of unregistered counsellors – there are some cowboys about.

The first session is usually an assessment to enable both you and your counsellor to see if you can work together. As counselling can cost £20–30 a session, make sure you feel comfortable. Ask as many questions as you like. The counsellor will certainly ask plenty of you to try to assess what you want and whether he or she can help.

A contract or programme may be used, which will include the goal of the counselling and the number of sessions that may be required to achieve it. Having a marker like this helps you keep sight of your target and reduces the chance of your going round and round in circles of hot air.

Many GP practices have counsellors associated with them, so it is well worth discussing the idea with your doctor.

PERSONAL DEVELOPMENT

Personal development takes self-management one step further. It addresses your whole life, not just your disease. Young Arthritis Care, who operate from the same address as Arthritis Care, run excellent personal development courses which change the lives of those who take them.

I have said elsewhere in this book that people are not so much disabled by their physical impairments, such as arthritis, but by others' attitudes to them and the inappropriate environment in which we live. If you're still feeling unconvinced by that, a personal development course could be the answer.

Courses are not yet widely available and those that are tend to be aimed at younger people. However, the range is increasing to include some targeted at people from minority communities and others for people who have retired. Contact Arthritis Care or your local rheumatology department for further information. These comments from Chris Helms are typical of those from participants:

'The personal development course was one of the best things I've ever done. I stopped seeing my problems as my fault. It helped me understand how it is society that disables us, not our individual impairments, however mild or severe they might be. It was very challenging – you've got to dig deep into yourself – but it's very exciting. I've developed skills that aren't just relevant to me because I've got arthritis but which everyone would benefit from – how to set personal goals, build self-confidence and so on. I know myself a lot better now. I'm no longer a poor little person – I'm perfectly capable and my views matter. Specifically, it's put me in the position to find work.

'I just didn't want to miss any of the course. It was so very positive. It turned my life around.'

SELF-HELP GROUPS

Self-help or support groups bring together people with arthritis to share ideas and experiences. They may be primarily social or more concerned with practical issues such as pain control. Some are led by people with arthritis themselves (often called 'user-led'), others by health professionals.

Arthritis Care has a network of more than 650 branches and local groups throughout the country. Some are user-led, particularly those targeted at younger people with arthritis. There are also groups for older people and some with a specifically Asian or Afro-Caribbean programme. Some concentrate on self-help, others on outings and social events. With a bit of luck you might be able to find a group suitable for you nearby. Contact Arthritis Care for more information.

You could also ask your doctor or consultant about local self-help – keep an eye on the notices in the waiting room.

Don't be put off by the idea of meeting other people with your disease, some of whom may have it more severely than you. If you do feel like this, acknowledge it but then think about what you are really saying – not just about other people with arthritis but about yourself too. Do you want others to be scared of you because you have arthritis?

Carmel Sayce was a bit apprehensive when she went to her first Young Arthritis Care meeting: 'To be honest, I went along to be nosy and find out what they did. I found myself talking to everyone. It was very beneficial to be with other people in a similar position to myself, all having some form of arthritis. I felt comfortable with everyone. They were all so lovely and friendly that I assumed they'd all been meeting for years but in fact, it was only the second get-together they'd ever had.

'Everyone understands the pain and frustrations I have felt. We have lots of laughs at these meetings, discussing our individual experiences of life.'

Finally, there are many, many smaller charities and support and self-help groups for people with specific types of arthritis. A full list of these appears in Chapter 13.

CHAPTER 9

Arthritis and the Body

Every doctor you've ever spoken to and every book on arthritis you've ever read has probably stressed the importance of exercise. Unfortunately, this one is no different.

Rather than resting your joints when you develop arthritis, it is even more important that you exercise them. Exercise protects against joint damage, keeps muscles and joints working and can help prevent disability. Unexercised joints lose muscle strength and can become more painful and more unstable.

Exercise can not only prevent further loss of joint function, it can help to regain some of that which has been lost. This takes time and a regular commitment.

What's more, exercise isn't only good for your arthritis. It helps protect against heart problems, osteoporosis and diabetes. It can reduce pain and increase stamina and energy levels. Mentally, it makes you feel good and helps with sleep and relaxation (remember this benefit if you think you are too tired to exercise). Feeling fit can increase self-confidence. You may even live longer.

As we have said many times, everyone with arthritis is different, and this is very true when it comes to exercise. Certain exercises may be particularly beneficial or wholly inappropriate for you and your arthritis so it is important to develop a customised programme with a health professional. Other aspects of the disease such as inflammation, the extreme fatigue associated with RA and lupus and the lower bone mass in osteoporosis will also affect an exercise programme. You need to discuss all this with your doctor or physiotherapist.

The purpose of this chapter therefore is to introduce the

different types of exercise rather than to prescribe particular ones. There are plenty of exercise books listed in Chapter 13.

Your exercise programme needn't involve going to an expensive or pretentious gymnasium. Nor need it be too time-consuming (just twenty minutes of relatively mild exercise three times a week and daily stretching will make a noticeable difference).

If you're overweight, exercise combined with a healthy diet (see Chapter 7) is much more likely to have long-term benefits than diet alone. And it's never too late to start. But do talk to your GP.

With all exercise, observe the two-hour rule. If you have more pain two hours after exercising than you did before you started, do less next time. The best times to exercise are when you have least pain and stiffness and when any medication is having its maximum effect.

How fit are you?
Take your pulse. The easiest place to find it is your wrist. Place the finger (not thumb) of the opposite hand just to the thumb side of the tendons running down the centre of your wrist. You should be able to feel the radial artery throbbing away. If you can't find it, ask your doctor to show you. Count the number of beats over a number of fifteen second periods, average them out and multiply the result by four to get your pulse rate per minute.

The average adult pulse is seventy-two beats per minute, but the ideal rate varies with age. In general, the lower your pulse, the fitter you are. Your doctor can tell you what a reasonable pulse rate for you should be.

Generally, young men in their twenties or thirties with pulses in the high eighties should be concerned about their fitness. Older men should be wary of a pulse over ninety. Women have higher pulse rates than men. A pulse close to 100 suggests a younger woman is unfit although for those over fifty, up to 102 is acceptable.

You can use your pulse to monitor your exercise programme. Your doctor can advise you what level to allow your pulse to reach in different activities and what your 'recovery rate' (how quickly you return to your normal level) should be.

Being fit involves stamina, co-ordination, strength, muscular endurance and suppleness. Different exercises develop different aspects of fitness. There are three basic types of exercise.

STRETCHING EXERCISES

Stretching, or range of movement (ROM) exercises involve moving the joint through its full range of movement and then just coaxing it a little bit further. Be gentle, don't force or jerk. These exercises are also very important as warm-ups for more energetic forms of exercise.

There are ROM exercises for the wrists and hands, the elbows, the shoulders, the neck, the spine, the hips, the knees and the feet and ankles.

Ideally each joint should be taken through its full ROM three to ten times and twice a day. Even inflamed joints should be gently eased through their ROM. This maintains joint range and may improve it over time.

In osteoarthritis, cartilage damage can be kept down by daily ROM exercises. Simply moving the joint squeezes the waste products out of the cartilage rather like water from a sponge. Cartilage will deteriorate if it is not exercised.

For rheumatoid arthritis these exercises may help with morning stiffness. Try them before rising or during your morning bath. Others find it helps to do them the night before, last thing before bed.

Stretching exercises are important for maintaining flexibility in ankylosing spondylitis. The Achilles' tendon (the cord in the back of the heel) is particularly at risk and must be kept supple.

STRENGTHENING EXERCISES

By tightening and releasing the muscles around a joint, these exercises can help restore strength in particular joints. Your physio or GP will tell you which joints you need to try these on and can also advise on the use of weights to make the muscles work harder.

Initially these exercises can be quite difficult. You may only be able to contract for a second or so. It will improve. Aim to hold for five to six seconds, relax, and repeat four times, twice a day. Strengthening exercises are not a substitute for stretching exercises – they develop the surrounding muscles, not range of movement. Particular strengthening exercises, along with stretching exercises, can be useful in improving posture.

ENDURANCE EXERCISE

This is the sort of thing we generally mean when we talk about taking exercise – activities such as walking, cycling, running, swimming, sport and so on. It is particularly important that you choose types of endurance exercise appropriate to your arthritis.

Endurance exercise should be aerobic. Literally this means 'requiring oxygen'. In practice it should leave you a little breathless and with an increased heart rate. Calculate your exercise heart rate by subtracting your age from 220. Multiply the result by 0·8 to find the maximum and by 0·6 to find the minimum. Try to exercise comfortably in this range. After five minutes of aerobic exercise take your pulse. If it is above the maximum, slow down.

Aerobic exercise burns off calories, increases the body's metabolism, reduces the levels of 'bad' cholesterol (LDL cholesterol) which can clog the arteries, and raises the levels of 'good' cholesterol (HDL cholesterol) which may prevent it.

If there is a concern about your blood cholesterol levels, your doctor may suggest a test before starting exercise, or you could ask for one. They can be done in the surgery. DIY kits from the pharmacists are generally less reliable. More about cholesterol on page 92.

Endurance exercise should last at least twenty minutes, three times a week.

All endurance exercise should be preceded with a warm-up and finish with a warm-down. To warm up, use a mixture of your personal stretching and strengthening exercises plus any particularly appropriate for the exercise you will be taking. To warm down, continue the aerobic exercise but in slow-motion – stroll after walking, pedal gently after cycling – and, to take advantage of your muscles' warmth, add in some gentle stretches.

Which endurance exercise is best depends on you and your arthritis. It is essential that you discuss this with your doctor. Here are some of the more popular ones with people with arthritis:

Walking

Walking three miles in an hour should burn off about 300 calories, walking five will burn off 480. Walking is a very cheap activity and you should be able to find opportunities to do it as part of your normal routine. Walk to the shops, office or round to a friend's. Unless you feel discomfort even over short distances, it is still possible to take up walking if you normally use a walking-stick. Again, discuss it with your GP.

Make sure you have shoes that are appropriate for you. Crepe, composite soles or training shoes tend to absorb the impact from the ground better than leather shoes. Insoles, available in most shoe shops or pharmacists, can be trimmed to size and will increase the support. Take your walking shoes with you when shopping for insoles.

Warm up for a brisk walk with a few minutes of gentle strolling. Warm down too. This should help you avoid strains. So will walking on a flat, level surface. Negotiating hills and uneven terrain increases pressure on your joints. Most importantly, find your own pace and enjoy it. Swinging your arms will help you burn off more calories.

Swimming

An hour's swimming can burn off between 350 and 750 calories, depending on what stroke you do and how quickly. Front crawl and butterfly are the most energetic, standing in the shallow end chatting to your friend the least.

Getting a Grip

Take it easy at first and change strokes regularly to exercise all your muscles. Take a hot shower afterwards.

Something that has really made a difference to me when swimming is to use a snorkel and mask. The neck movements involved in breathing for breast-stroke and crawl were painful for me. With the snorkel and mask I have no need to move my head at all. It takes a bit of getting used to but it can add to the fun, especially if you enjoy swimming underwater. Check if your local pool allows them. Because of the potential danger to children, mine only allows them in adult-only sessions.

The sides of a pool can be very slippery, so you might want to invest in some appropriate rubber-soled footwear.

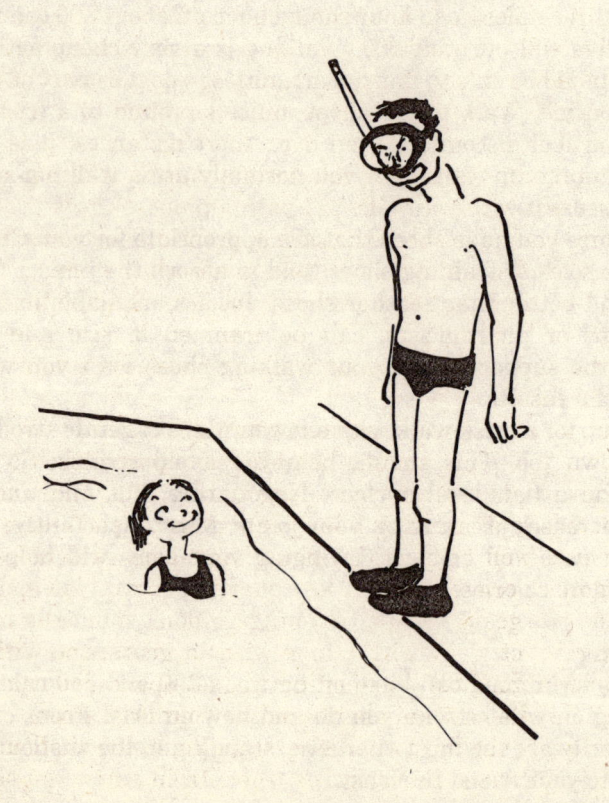

It is easier to exercise in water than on dry land because the water takes much of the weight of your body. You can do more with less pain. That is why Aquarobics and other water-based exercises classes are becoming more popular. Your doctor or physiotherapist may be able to refer you to a hydrotherapy clinic for specialist treatment in a lovely warm pool. Or you can join a local group.

Ideally, pool temperatures for exercise should be around eighty-four degrees Fahrenheit, although most local swimming pools are nearer 80–83. It's worth bearing this in mind if you are sensitive to the cold. Make sure the trainer is qualified and knows something about arthritis. Find out about Aquarobics – which is water-based aerobic exercise – in your area. Make sure you don't overdo it. Speaking from personal experience, it's very easy to do.

Cycling
Cycling at 12mph uses up 600 calories an hour. It is rather more expensive to take up than walking or swimming, so check that it's for you. Talk to your doctor and to other cyclists. Try to have a go either on a friend's bike or ask in your local cycling store.

Cycling can keep you fit, get you from A to B and provide a great way to see the countryside. However, it is dangerous. Falling off, especially in the city, is an ever-present risk for even the most experienced cyclist. If you physically would be unable to take a fall, or if balance, vision or hearing impairments might make one more likely, cycling is probably not appropriate.

Your arthritis can affect your choice of bike. You might fancy the lighter frame of a racing bike, but the drop handle-bars, for instance, may well be out. Get the handle-bars replaced with something more comfortable. A key question is, can you operate the brakes and gears? While, if your legs don't mind the extra work, you can get away with a bike without gears, one without brakes is not a good idea! Adjusting the set-up or layout of the brakes and handle-bars may help – ask at your local store.

Make sure you use the correct size cycle. Your elbows should be comfortably bent and the back free from strain when you sit on

Getting a Grip

the saddle and hold the handle-bars. To check the height, put your heel on the pedal and push it down. When the pedal is at its lowest point, your leg should be straight. If it's still bent the seat is too low and you will strain your knees. If the seat is too high, you can strain your back.

When actually cycling use the ball of your foot and wear a helmet.

Static cycling
You can burn up just as many calories without ever leaving your house. A decent static bike or exercise cycle can cost as much as a regular bicycle but there are no awkward brakes or gears to operate and no chance of falling off.

Some features you might find include a speedometer, a mileometer and calorie counter. The more hi-tech types found in health clubs and gyms can provide a variety of computerised terrains for you to cycle over and they even take your pulse afterwards. You can often adjust the pedal resistance to suit you, and the number of calories you want to expend every hour.

All these gadgets make it much easier to chart your progress than with regular cycling. Use your journal to record times, distances and calories shed.

The guidance for choosing a road cycle also applies to choosing a static bike.

The problem with static cycling is boredom. The only scenery is the mantelpiece. Solutions include:

★ watching TV – I use my exercise bike as an excuse to catch up on the soap operas. There are even videos available full of exciting scenery rushing past as seen from the cyclists' viewpoint!
★ listening to music
★ reading – you can get book racks to clip on to the handlebars.

Whichever kind of cycling you choose, start slowly and don't do it for too long. The muscles used in cycling are different to those used in walking and some may be a little out of practice. Work up to your targets.

Other gymnasium equipment
There is a vast range of exercise machines available. Walking, running, rowing, skiing – you name it, there is a machine that simulates it. Take a look in your local gym. They're not cheap, but one might be particularly helpful to you. Talk to your doctor.

Sports
There are also, of course, many sports that you can try out, from low-impact aerobics (no jumping) to high-impact rugby union! If you find exercising alone dull, competitive sports can be more sociable. Ask your doctor what he or she would suggest. Golf, if you walk and carry your clubs, burns off between 300 and 600 calories an hour, depending on whether you're playing on the municipal pitch-and-putt or at St Andrew's. Ballroom dancers expend 360 calories an hour, tennis players 480, aerobics enthusiasts 360–480 and squash players up to 900.

EVERYDAY EXERCISE

We all know a healthy, balanced diet is much better for us than periods of overeating followed by crash diets, and it's much the same with exercise. A generally active life will keep you fitter and healthier than months of indolence followed by a week in the gym. Everyday activities do burn off calories and strengthen and stretch your muscles. But think about them much as you might an exercise – that is:

★ try to do them properly – lift with the knees not the back, sit up straight and so on, and
★ adapt them to make them suitable for you – more about this in Chapter 11.

Vacuuming burns off 250 calories an hour, driving 168, and cleaning the windows 300. Even standing (108) and sleeping (78) burn some calories. However, this does not mean that having a kip can now be legitimately termed a form of exercise.

CHAPTER 10

Arthritis and Others

Good relationships with other people begin with a good relationship with yourself. Positive self-esteem is important to all aspects of living with arthritis, but it's in the area of personal relationships where you can really start to enjoy your feelings of self-worth. And so can other people.

When I planned this book, the idea was that there would be sections on your partner, the rest of your family, your friends, and the rest of the world! However, as I began to write it, I was repeating myself over and over again because, whatever the relationship, the key to success is in honest communication.

As one woman with arthritis said: 'The most important thing – and also the most difficult – in any relationship, is to talk about your needs, likes and dislikes.' So I've concentrated instead on what you can do to be an honest communicator. Of course you will treat your children differently to your parents, but the principle should be the same.

For a book on sex and relationships, look no further than Young Arthritis Care's *Our Relationships, Our Sexuality*. I am grateful to Penny Boot (a.k.a. Kata Kolbert), the title's main author, for many of the ideas in this chapter.

ONLY YOU UNDERSTAND

To someone with arthritis, it goes without saying that only people with arthritis really know what the disease is like. Even the most understanding of your family or friends – people you see every day of your life – don't really know. The problem is that so many people think they do. In most cases, it's not arrogance, it's ignorance. Not that it's their fault.

They think they know because of what they've seen and heard. In the media, there are two images of arthritis. The first, reflecting the fact that many people have the disease, is the idea that it is something trivial that happens to old people. The second, arising out of the media's general stereotype of disabled people, is that it is something terrible that leaves you in a wheelchair and dependent.

It's very confusing. And very inaccurate. On one hand, arthritis is never trivial, and on the other, using a wheelchair does not mean giving up your independence. In fact, I don't know anybody who fits into either of these stereotypes.

Images of pity
Images in the media and those used by charities to raise money turn everybody with a disability into a victim or a hero. The media particularly like the heroes – people who have triumphed over their disability, achieved despite it. They make what journalists call good 'human interest' stories and sell newspapers. Examples involving people with arthritis include the woman who climbed Everest, the boy who got a degree, the girl who does ballet and the man who ran a marathon. At best these stories are patronising; at worst they read like a Victorian freak-show. They all dwell on the strangeness of difference.

Meanwhile, the charities prefer the victims – pathetic individuals whose lives will be worthless without your pennies. People whose bodies, in one charity advertising campaign, are literally torn apart. Funny how a few coppers can turn you from victim to hero.

It's no wonder that people are so scared of x disease or y impairment. They know they're just regular people. They know they couldn't be heroes, so if they got whatever it is, they think they'd wind up victims. Perhaps that's how you felt when you were first diagnosed. On diagnosis of arthritis, people often swing wildly from imagining the worst possible scenario to totally ignoring and belittling their condition – after all, if you don't feel like a hero or a victim then perhaps you haven't really got it. Of course, as someone with arthritis, you come to know it's all nonsense. Most people with disabilities are neither heroes nor victims, they are just regular people who happen to have x or y.

The effect of these images is to put a barrier between people with a disability – whether it be arthritis, HIV or a broken spine – and people without. A lot of the problems associated with what people sometimes call 'coming to terms' with your disability arise from trying to square your own perceptions of what it's like on the other side of the barrier with what you know about yourself. Once you realise that the people on the other side of the barrier are just the same as the people on 'your' side, the barrier simply disappears.

However, although the barrier might disappear for you, it will still be there for others. That is why honest communication is vital for people with arthritis. This is the best way you can help others to remove the barrier. Such communication is difficult at the best of times, and impossible if you cannot find at your core a strong sense of your own self-worth.

BUILDING SELF-ESTEEM

In the face of the media pressure outlined above, it is small wonder that building self-esteem is so difficult. It involves:

★ accepting your arthritis so that, for you, the barrier can disappear
★ recognising that, if the barrier will not disappear for others, it is down to their ignorance and is their problem

Both these things are easier said than done.

Arthritis is even more difficult to accept if you already have a low opinion of yourself. You may feel inadequate physically – too fat, too thin, big nose – or intellectually – not clever – or socially – not fun to be with. If you already feel like this and have arthritis, it is doubly difficult. After all, the physical effects of arthritis do not form part of the media and advertising industry's diktats about the body beautiful.

Overcoming low self-esteem is a very real problem for many, many people, not just those with arthritis, and saying that it can be overcome is not to minimise the difficulty of doing it. Whether you can do this yourself or with family or friends, or need the help of someone else such as a counsellor or therapist, is something only you can decide. This book cannot give you self-confidence. Only you can. What can help?

★ Talking to other people with arthritis, particularly those of your own age and sex.
★ Personal development courses can make a massive difference.
★ Taking time out for yourself to think about what you want – just giving yourself this little bit of self-respect can be a great start.
★ Reading this book and others that take a positive approach to living with arthritis and affirm your right to enjoy it.

When people around you, particularly those you love, have a problem with your arthritis, it is very difficult to accept that it is their problem not yours. For the woman who said, 'I have problems with my self-image mainly due to parental attitude. They were never able to accept that I would be able to have an adult relationship as they were never able to accept my disability,' the first step to positive self-esteem was leaving home. Not easy.

COMMUNICATION

When you feel comfortable with yourself, it is much easier to communicate with others. Only through your communicating honestly can they overcome their misconceptions and ignorance about arthritis.

Penny Boot says: 'Sadly, it must be acknowledged that some partnerships and relationships will not last through the pressures of your developing arthritis. What is important is that the person with arthritis does not allow feelings of guilt and rejection to swamp their self-worth when this happens, as it may well be failings within the able-bodied person that caused it. Blame should not fall automatically to you because you feel your arthritis must be blamed for everything.'

This is true of relationships with lovers, with friends and with family.

Building on a base of your own self-worth, communication skills and assertiveness can be developed. Many people with arthritis have found courses in both of these very useful, particularly with other people with arthritis. They both involve being honest – with yourself about what you want and with others. Sugaring the pill with humour is great if you can manage it, but don't be manipulative. Being 'brave' and expecting someone else 'to notice' is being manipulative. So is playing on others' good nature or guilt.

As a person with arthritis, you have a right to challenge behaviour that you find inappropriate just as anyone has, but focus on the behaviour rather than the person doing it. Some tips for positive communication:

★ acknowledge how you feel
★ don't apologise for yourself or how you feel
★ don't beat about the bush or flatter or patronise
★ if you give a reason for a request, make sure it's genuine

Sometimes you might need to think about exactly how you do this depending on who you are dealing with. Obviously children have their own needs and wants which you will want to acknowledge. For example, if you can't give your son a piggy-back because your back hurts say so, but you might want to clarify that it's not because you don't want to.

MAKING LOVE

One aspect of our personal relationships where the need for honest communication is even greater is with our sexual partners.

As one person with arthritis said: 'Nothing kills sex more than saying "that hurt". I tend to point out the problem areas in advance but this needs confidence and trust in your partner. Nothing beats a permanent relationship when the qualities can mature.'

Penny Boot says: 'Work on being assertive enough to tell your partner what hurts you, without making it sound like an out-and-out rejection, and also be clear about what you find particularly pleasurable. A loving partner will never make you feel guilty about being in pain.'

Again there can be a tendency to blame arthritis for any shortcomings in the bedroom. Being honest with yourself and your partner will help you assess how far this is true. You may find you agree with this woman: 'I don't feel that all the sexual problems in the relationships that haven't been so good were caused by arthritis – they are often caused by different problems.'

Sex is to be enjoyed, and you have this right. 'With communication, you and your partner can set about exploring new ways to make love, ways which should be pleasurable – and fun – to both,' says Penny.

Avoid any position which is immediately painful. Take your time; sex does not have to be focused on penetration and orgasm. A slower approach to sex, with rests, can heighten excitement and pleasure. You may need to experiment, which can be fun for both partners. The best time for making love is when you feel least pain – after painkillers, for example.

Practically, sex toys and aids can be great if your fingers aren't so nimble. For the same reason, it is a good idea to unwrap condoms in advance! If you experience vaginal dryness, as is often the case with lupus or Sjogren's syndrome, use a water-based lubricant such as K-Y jelly. It is best kept to a minimum in the vagina with a small layer applied directly to the penis. Oil-based lubricants can damage vaginal tissue and also condoms.

Some lovemaking positions recommended by people with arthritis are:

★ Spoons – man lies behind woman and enters from there. 'A very gentle position and suitable for people who have difficulties in most joints.'

★ Crossways – man lies on his side and woman lies perpendicularly across him, bottom touching his lower thigh, her vagina meeting his penis side on. Her legs can bend over his body or be kept straight using a cushion. 'One you can do for hours, although one or both partners will need to be able to roll back and forward during sex.'

★ Rear entry – woman lies on stomach supported by cushions or whatever; man lies over top of her and, supporting own weight, enters vagina from behind. 'Many variations are possible as long as you lose your inhibitions about it.'

★ Woman on top – good when man has arthritis.

All these positions are discussed in more detail and with illustrations in *Our Relationships, Our Sexuality*. There are also many variations on the missionary for you to discover. Penny Boot says: 'Any of these positions can be varied to suit your needs. It is best to approach new methods light-heartedly.'

You needn't think your partner is doing you a favour by allowing all this – far from it. You can guarantee them that they will enjoy it too once they lose any inhibitions they may have.

One non-disabled journalist in his thirties says the need to communicate has enabled his relationship with his wife (who has arthritis) to flourish. He has some excellent advice for other non-disabled partners: 'You need to be able to communicate needs both general and sexual and to share responsibilities as you see fit. People in traditional male–female partnership roles may find this difficult, but change is always possible.

'Always ask about how to give help. Don't assume. It may be something as simple as moving something or helping them lift a heavy glass down the pub. It may be something like finding a sexual position where your partner is completely comfortable. If these things bother you or cause you worry or embarrassment about not being right or normal, then it is probably you who needs to challenge your way of thinking.

'Problems can be overcome if you actually talk to each other and tackle changes positively. Of course a great side-effect of this is a genuine closeness, emotionally and physically – something that many non-disabled couples spend their lives searching for.'

Much of what has been said already applies equally to non-heterosexual relationships. The gay scene – particularly for males – suffers from similarly rigid notions of physical beauty.

For some, the 'double difference' of being gay and disabled can make it easier. For some it can make it harder. Having one difference may make it easier to deal with having another one. On the other hand, the challenge of one difference may be enough.

Some lesbians, like many disabled women, shun the stereotypically beautiful feminine look. 'In this respect,' said one lesbian with arthritis, 'it might be a little easier to fit in as a disabled lesbian than as a disabled heterosexual woman.'

For further information and useful contacts see the directory section.

CHAPTER 11

Arthritis at Home and Work

There are many aids and gadgets that people with arthritis can use to make everyday tasks easier – from a chunky foam grip making a pen easier to hold to a voice-operated computer, from an automatic tin-opener to a fully adapted low-level kitchen, from a grab-rail in the bathroom to a wheelchair. You may use many or none.

The fact that there are so many possibilities only serves to prove the point that it is not arthritis that causes disability, but the environment in which we live.

For me, the discovery that there are computers that can be trained to recognise your voice (and that they work) has been a career-saver. Whatever you do, the objective is to protect your joints enabling you to do more more easily.

When you have arthritis, you become an excellent planner – a skill that is very valuable at home and work. You also become very resourceful. Many people talk of how their resourcefulness and creativity was liberated when they stopped seeing the problems arising from their arthritis as their fault or as something to be ashamed of and to hide.

In the case of my repetitive strain injury, it's not that I can't write or use a word-processor, it is that the standard word-processor with a keyboard is, for me, badly designed. (In fact, the standard QWERTY keyboard is badly designed for everyone; the original purpose of the layout of the keys on a manual typewriter was to slow typists down so that the keys did not lock – but that's another story.) Rather than give up using the word-processor, I looked around for a solution – a different way of word-processing.

Getting a Grip

With modern technology moving at the pace it is, it's amazing how many problems can be solved.

Don't get me wrong – this wasn't easy or quick. It took me a long time to get there. It took me a long time and a fair bit of self-loathing to realise that the problem was not with me but with the computer. Once I did, the problem became one that could be solved.

Knowing someone who has already solved the problem, as I did, made an enormous difference, but there are still feelings and emotions that you have to go through for yourself.

WHAT THINGS ARE DIFFICULT FOR YOU?

Whatever it is, the problem is not in you, it's in the environment, the things around you. Things like my computer. And the good thing about the environment is that, like my computer, it can be changed. This chapter looks at some of the things that can be done at home and work.

Solving problems involves using one or more of the following four approaches – you probably do this every day already.

★ Changing the way that a task is performed – for example, protecting your hands by carrying things to work in a shoulder bag or satchel rather than a briefcase.
★ Adapting the environment to make the task easier – this can range from putting a non-slip mat in the bath or shower to having a wall knocked down.
★ Buying a new gadget or adaptation.
★ Inventing a new gadget – your own devices custom-built to your own specifications by yourself or a willing friend.

Kate Lorig's *Arthritis Helpbook* has an excellent chapter on this subject. It identifies the specific dos and don'ts involved in making a task easier.

★ Distribute the load over strong joints or a larger area – for

example, using the hand to operate an aerosol rather than just the finger, using your hip to close a drawer, etc . . .
★ Use body leverage – hold things as close to the body as possible.
★ Avoid holding the same joint position for long periods – stretch frequently, change your position.
★ Try to keep a good posture – when sitting, standing, lifting, etc.

She advocates an eight-point approach to problem solving.

★ Identify the problem – for example, I couldn't use my word-processor.
★ Pinpoint what causes it – pushing the keys hurt.
★ Make a list of possible solutions – write by hand; dictate to someone; find another job/stop writing; find a suitable word-processor.
★ Choose one – find a suitable word-processor.
★ Research it – approached specialist disability computing consultants; talked to others in similar position.
★ Assess it – tried one version on loan.
★ If it fails choose another – worked well, but hardware not entirely suitable for my type of work.
★ Assess it – at time of writing awaiting chance to try alternative.

And so on until a solution emerges. When selecting items and gadgets:

★ Those with wheels should be easier to move than those without.
★ The longer the lever the better – products employing the benefits of the lever principle will be easier to use than those that do not. To see what a big difference it makes, put a knife under the ring-pull on a can and use that as a lever. Compare it with opening the can normally.
★ Think about weight – plastic and aluminium culinary items are lighter than stoneware or Pyrex; nylon or canvas bags will be lighter than leather ones.

★ Look at the size of the grip or handle – in theory the bigger it is, the easier it is to hold (within reason!).

★ As far as possible exploit technology – opt for labour-saving gadgets such as food-processors, blenders, microwaves, stay-pressed clothing and so on.

★ Shop around. There are specialist suppliers of disability products but in fact, many of the labour-saving devices aimed at the public in general are particularly useful for people with arthritis and often cheaper than the 'specialist' items.

★ If possible try before you buy. Can you reach and operate all the controls properly? If you're buying an electric tin-opener, for example, take some empty tins with you and try the various models out on the bottom end of the cans. Any decent store should happily allow this.

★ For more expensive items such as washing machines, spin driers, dishwashers and so on, it might be worth hiring rather than buying straight away to check that the product is for you.

If, at the end of Chapter 3, you made a list of the specific problems that your arthritis brings, you could, when you've finished this chapter, have a go at applying Kate Lorig's eight-point plan to them.

ARTHRITIS AT HOME

How you organise your home obviously depends on a lot of factors including how much room you have, who else you live with and how you like to spend your time. These are just some ideas. You can probably think of more. And, don't forget, if you can think of a gadget, you can probably buy it – somewhere.

The kitchen
Margaret Lees, who is an Arthritis Care self-help trainer, gave me some tips on how to organise your kitchen for easier cooking.

★ Two easier ways to boil rice, pasta, vegetables or potatoes:

– for small quantities use a milk pan – they're lighter.

– for larger quantities use a wire mesh basket (from a deep-fat fryer, perhaps) in the saucepan and boil in that. After cooking, simply removing the basket from the saucepan drains the food immediately and the basket is much easier to manoeuvre than a heavy water-filled saucepan.

★ Cook items together to save working with a number of pans – add the peas when the potatoes are half-cooked, for example.

★ Make sure everything is at the right level for you. Margaret says: 'I now use a combination oven/microwave/grill which sits on the work-surface. This allows me to cook whatever I like without any need to bend or stretch. As I'm only four foot eight I'd need a periscope to use the conventional "eye-level" grill! I also keep the things I need on the top shelf of the fridge.' Maximise storage space at your optimum working level by using storage boxes and racks. Keep flour, sugar and the like in scoop-out containers to save lifting jars or bags.

★ Cook more when you can – on good days, when your arthritis isn't feeling too bad, cook more than you need and freeze it in single-serving size containers. Then, on a day when you're not feeling so good, shove one of these in the microwave.

★ Be safe – securing vegetables on a spiked chopping board will allow you to slice, chop or peel them without having to hold them steady in your other hand.

★ Use the kitchen drawer to open packets – open a drawer and place the uncooperative packet of biscuits or whatever upright in it. Shut the drawer so that the packet is held tight and open it with a knife or scissors. Something similar may be possible in order to secure a small bowl for mixing. But be careful.

★ Make washing up easier – ideally, get someone else to do it (some hope!), but if this is not possible put pans and dishes in to soak in warm water as quickly as possible after using them. After washing up don't waste energy drying them, just let them drain.

Gadgets that you can buy for the kitchen include large-handled cutlery; tippers and pourers for teapots and kettles; slicing guides to help with cutting bread or cake; 'grip-mats' for opening bottles

Getting a Grip

and jars; lever-taps and other devices for making taps easier to operate; similar items for cookers and gas-taps.

The bathroom
This is an important room. You can't avoid it for long, and a long relaxing bath can do more for you than just keep you clean. However, slippery floors and the lack of space in the typical bathroom can make them difficult to negotiate. Advance planning of the operation becomes particularly important.

A bath board, which goes across the bath, or a bath seat, which fits inside it, can make getting in and out easier. Some electrically operated hoists and lifts can actually lower you in and out of the bath. A rubberised non-slip mat makes standing safer. Grab-rails correctly affixed and positioned – talk to an occupational therapist – may also help. Again, lever-style taps are available.

A shower may be easier for you to use. It may not be so relaxing but it can be very invigorating.

Gadgets which some people have found useful when washing include sponges and brushes with long handles, broad-handled or electric toothbrushes and liquid soap dispensers.

To make your toilet more accessible, a raised seat may make all the difference. Grab-rails or a surround frame (which is attached to the floor and sits around the toilet a little like a walking frame) can also help.

Around the home
Plugs and sockets: There are a number of ways of making sockets more accessible without actually rewiring: an extension lead (beware of trailing cable) or a powerpoint raiser, which attaches to the wall and raises the socket (not elegant but safer), can be used in tandem with moulded plug handles or the cheaper detachable plug-pullers which make it easier to remove the plugs from the sockets.
Chairs: Try to have at least one chair which really suits you: comfortable to sit in and easy to rise from. If you can achieve this, any money invested – for example, on a reclining model – is

probably money well spent. To help, the ARC produce a useful booklet called *Are You Sitting Comfortably*. For example, block-raisers which attach to the legs are available to raise the height of a chair or bed.

Think about how you get up and sit down. Use your weight to your advantage rather than support it all on your arms and hands to push yourself up. Rock your head and body forward from the waist and use the momentum to help you up. The Alexander Technique (see page 72) specifically looks at sitting and rising properly.

Beds: Most people with arthritis will benefit from a firmer bed. A loose, sagging one puts strain on the joints. This needn't be a specialist 'orthopaedic' model. Try it in the shop. A wooden base with legs may be better than a divan, as block-raisers can then be attached if required.

Utilities: The electricity, telephone and gas companies should be able to provide a leaflet with information about their special services for disabled people or even a personal adviser. They are usually keen to help.

Grippers, grabbers and extending gizmos

Grabbers, reachers and other extension-type gadgets are very popular. Margaret Lees has developed her own multi-purpose 'hook stick' – it's a pole with a hook screwed on the end (total cost around 40p). She uses it for taking clothes out of the washing machine, for pulling on her trousers, closing the tailgate of her hatchback car, turning switches on and off and so on. She also attaches a duster to it for dusting and a roller or paintbrush for decorating. Margaret says: 'That's the beauty of making your own gadgets – once they're made, there's no end to the uses you can find for them.' Perhaps the cheapest and easiest to make DIY extension gizmo is the bent metal coathanger.

Long-arm gripper products for picking up items from the floor or getting them on and off a shelf are also widely available in the shops. Some have a magnet on the end for reclaiming pins and needles. Others are designed to aid dressing. One of these could be just what you need, but do try before you buy and, as with any purchase but particularly with a specialist 'disability' item, shop around. Prices can vary considerably.

'There are catalogues available which sell special gadgets for disabled people. For many who buy them they work well but for others they may be too expensive or not suitable to the individual's physical abilities,' says Margaret Lees. 'I bought a reaching hand a few years ago for £30 but found my hand was too small to reach the trigger to work it properly. I then made my hook stick, and it does many more jobs than the reaching stick was designed to do.'

Housework

Many of us have been brought up to be house proud; having a clean and tidy house is as important as ourselves and our children being clean and tidy. When you have arthritis, it is necessary to look at this belief more objectively. It is *your* home – organise it to suit you. People who judge a person by the shine of their doorstep are the sort of people who judge a book by the cover.

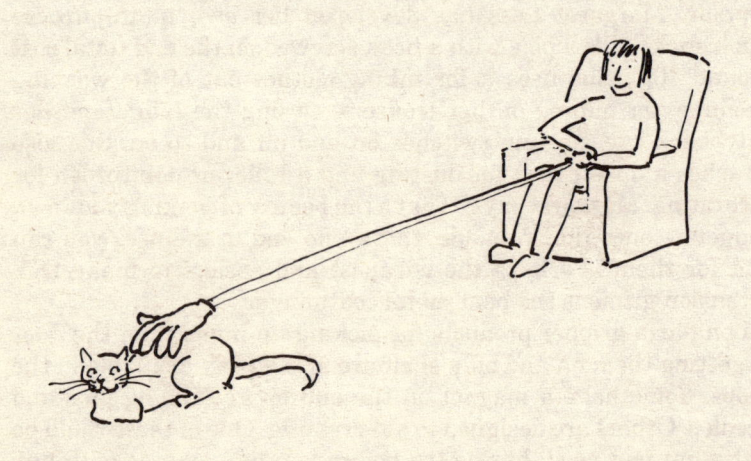

Look at what tasks really need to be done and how often. Unless you have a house-dust allergy, it is probably not necessary to vacuum and dust daily. Again, shop around for designs that work for you – height-adjustable ironing boards so you can sit down to iron, lightweight vacuum cleaners or hand-held ones for smaller jobs, self-cleaning ovens, self-defrosting fridges and so on. Iron only what really needs to be ironed.

Help in the home
If you need assistance with housework, help with buying special equipment or an adaptation made to your house, contact your local authority. They should be able to assist you under Community Care (see page 45). There are also volunteer agencies who may be able to provide a suitable helper, although this obviously is more of a lottery.

Adapting your home
Sometimes altering the fabric of your house might be the solution. Obviously nobody enters into this lightly but if you wish to look into it, your local authority planning department may be able to give advice. Unless you are planning on increasing the size of the property you should not need planning permission. Under the

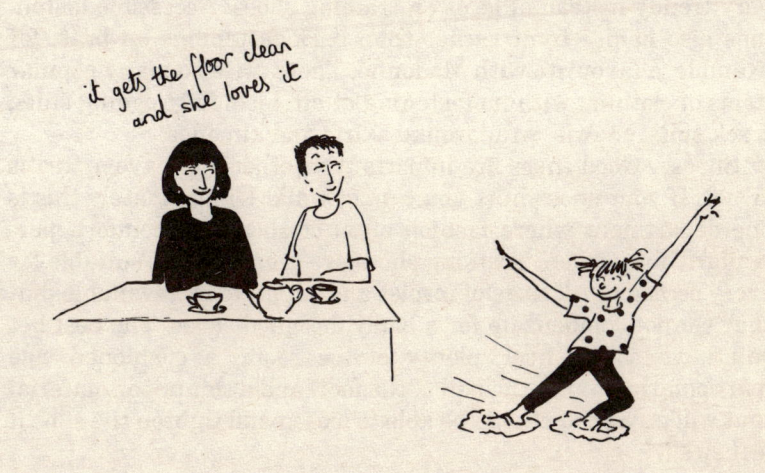

1990 Local Government and Housing Act limited house renovation grants are available. There are a number of types including a disabled facilities grant. They are all means-tested. Age Concern is a useful source of further information.

Clothing

With clothing, a bit of ingenuity goes a long way. With such a variety of fabrics, fastenings and styles to choose from it's usually possible to find something you feel good wearing and that you can actually get into. And think laterally. Why struggle with a tie when you can buy a clip-on? If you can't get a good loose fit in your size, buy larger sizes. Women, check out the men's department.

There are a number of specialist clothing companies, many of them operating by catalogue which, while increasing the likelihood of choosing an unsuitable garment, can take the hassle out of shopping.

★ Fastenings – Bigger buttons are usually easier than smaller ones. Similarly, the bigger the tab on the zip the easier it is to move – attaching a cord can also help. Velcro, with its hundreds of tiny fibre hooks, is particularly easy to use and, at the moment, very trendy instead of laces on training shoes. Accessible fastenings also help – front rather than back fastenings on bras, for example, a favourite with Madonna. There are also many popular items of clothing with no fastening at all, including jogging suits, track suits, shawls, wraparound skirts and kimonos.

★ Shoes – Good shoes are important whether you have arthritis or not. If your shoes hurt you cannot walk. Unfortunately this is one department where fashion often clashes with comfort, particularly for women. Training shoes are great but not suitable for every occasion. All sorts of insoles and supports are available, but they cannot compensate for a badly designed shoes. The best bet will have a low heel, plenty of toe room, a cushioned sole (particularly around the ball of the foot) and a soft upper material that will give. You should be able to loosen and tighten the shoe if feet swell.

If you have specialist footwear needs, discuss them with your *one merely holds the magnet THUS drawing the metal toggle irresistibly towards it, and thereby facilitating the undoing of my jacket*

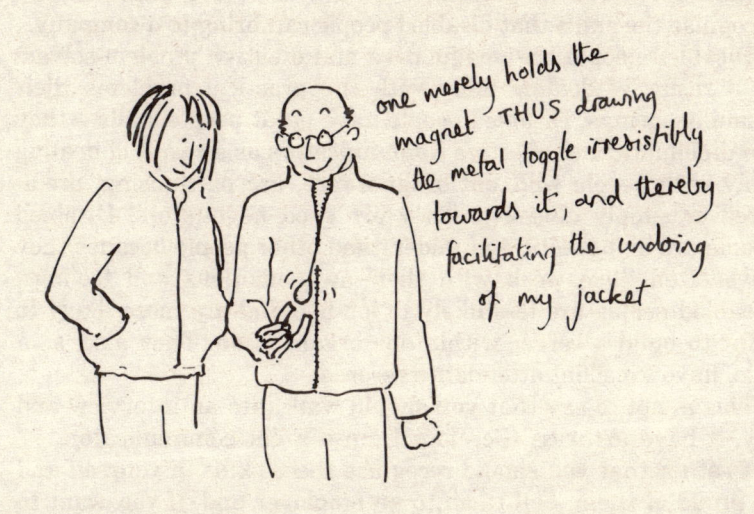

doctor who may be able to refer you to an orthotist or podiatrist – the NHS do supply orthopaedic footwear.

ARTHRITIS AT WORK

This section on work is in the same chapter as the section on the home because, in theory, similar adaptations and aids are available to make life easier for the person with arthritis. There's even the possibility of the Government paying for them! (More about that later.) In fact, there are considerable problems to overcome if you are actually to make this happen. If you are working, you'll know exactly what I mean. But take heart, the situation is improving.

First the good news. Traditionally, a disability at work has been something to be hidden, not to be talked of. It has, probably correctly, been regarded as reducing your chances of recruitment or promotion. In the 1990s, this attitude is changing. The more enlightened employers – which tend to be the larger ones with money to invest in personnel initiatives – are beginning to recognise the skills that disabled people can bring to a company.

Disabled people are imaginative and creative problem-solvers as a result of dealing daily with the practical problems their disability brings. Disabled people have great people skills – they are diplomatic and effective communicators as a result of dealing daily with people who, out of ignorance, are patronising, prejudiced or simply offensive. They are good negotiators. Disabled people are empathetic and understand other people because they have often done work with their own emotions and feelings. Disabled people are less likely to job-hop and are more likely to want to build a career within one organisation. They also, as a rule, have excellent attendance records.

This is not to say that you should walk into an interview and say, 'I have arthritis therefore I am a great communicator . . .' but rather that you should recognise these skills in yourself and be proud of them. Sell them to an employer and, if you want to draw on how your experience of disability has helped you develop them, don't be afraid to do so.

However, changes like this don't happen overnight; some employers will always be bigoted and in a time of recession personnel and recruitment policies will not be at the top of a manager's agenda. There are still real problems around arthritis in the workplace.

Disabled workers are less likely to be appointed in the first place than non-disabled candidates (unemployment among disabled people is about twice the national average), and less likely to be in managerial and professional grades. A survey by Excel Employment, a specialist recruitment agency for disabled people, found that only 6% of disabled workers were in these senior grades compared with 23% of non-disabled workers. This was despite the fact that many disabled people actually had better qualifications then their non-disabled colleagues and many were over-qualified for the posts they held. Fewer than one in five of the disabled people questioned felt their promotion prospects were good.

The problem is that old chestnut: ignorance. Employers don't understand arthritis any more or less than the rest of the population, but the fear that arises out of their ignorance is often more stark: they are terrified that it is going to cost them money. This is what some people whose arthritis has affected their work had to say:

Going it alone
'Many people with arthritis can live for years with the illness and yet show no outward signs. This apparent healthiness prevents the public from understanding the very real pain experienced with arthritis. Most people equate disability with wheelchairs. The various nuances of disability remain a mystery and this communication difficulty, I am certain, is one of the central reasons that people with arthritis have difficulty getting and keeping a job,' says a freelance journalist who opted to take advantage of all the government-sponsored small business initiatives to set up as self-employed. He finds he's able to 'mix and match' his work to suit the cyclical nature of arthritis.

Freelance working is becoming more popular – employers like it because it provides them with a more flexible work-force, and many freelancers enjoy the freedom to design their office to suit them, schedule their own workloads, choose their own hours and so on. As new technology develops, making it easier to work from home, and as commuting becomes ever more unpleasant, it will become an increasingly attractive option for those whose work makes it possible. Would self-employment help you? Discuss the option with a Disability Employment Adviser (see Access To Work below) or talk to your local Job Centre. You may get help, particularly if you are currently unemployed.

A not-so-voluntary redundancy
Years of training are no protection against discrimination. Highly trained professionals such as teachers can also encounter ignorant and unimaginative employers.

'When newly diagnosed after being in terrific pain for about a year, I told my headteacher that I needed a hip replacement. His answer was, "Oh." On a couple of occasions I mentioned the difficulties I was experiencing teaching the younger children, but no offer was made to relieve me. The head didn't like teaching infants. The really upsetting part was my head saying I was disruptive to the school. He was totally insensitive. The children had supply teachers, and they were people who had covered while I had been on courses so the children knew them. They didn't appear to be missing out. Eventually I was so poorly I had to be long-term sick and, just prior to my hip operation, I got early retirement on health grounds. I'd had no support from my head to stay in the profession and never once were my employers, the county council, approached to see if they could have offered me something else.'

This ex-primary school teacher is now a self-help trainer for a voluntary organisation. She recommends voluntary work as a way back.

'Voluntary work often leads to other things. Meeting people and talking helps. For me, the thing is to keep busy in whatever area you feel comfortable and, hopefully, it will help your situation. What works for one doesn't always work for another, but no matter how dark the days can get, keep exploring different avenues and eventually it'll pay off. It has for me.'

Volunteering is a growth area. If you fancy it, get in touch with your local volunteer bureau. Their number should be under Voluntary Services in the local Thomson directory. Volunteering should not make any difference to any welfare benefits you might be on, but do check. There's more about benefits on page 157.

Inflexible 'friends'

It doesn't matter how honest you are about your arthritis if your colleagues just aren't prepared to alter their familiar way of doing things. This applies even with a local authority, who are generally, because of their size and political commitment to serving the whole community, more enlightened employers.

'I accepted a job working as a clerical assistant for a local authority and stressed at the interview that I had limitations caused by rheumatoid arthritis. Upon commencing, I soon discovered that I was expected to make tea and coffee for the rest of the staff, carrying a heavy tray laden with pot, cups and saucers. I was also expected to do something known as the "Bun Run", which involved dashing across a busy road armed with carrier bags to do daily shopping for staff lunches. In all weathers. I was told to travel once a week in a taxi, delivering post to forty schools only to discover that I was expected to carry each package and personally deliver it to the school. I was unable to do this and was told by the taxi driver that he was not insured to carry anything. Fortunately he took pity on me and agreed to help just once. It was obvious to me that I could not continue the duties required from this job and handed in my notice.'

It is hard to see any of these duties as essential to the post. They could have been done by anyone. In fact, sharing these tasks would probably have made for a happier office.

Should you tell your boss?

Because of these attitudes, most people with arthritis are unsure whether to tell employers or potential employers about their disease. There are advantages and disadvantages to both – you will have to make your own decision based on your situation.

Advantages of telling

★ Employer could change your work or adjust your role to make it easier for you.
★ Specialist equipment may be available either from your employer or from the state (see Access To Work on page 155), or you may simply choose to bring something for yourself from home.
★ Colleagues who know can become colleagues who understand.
★ It is hard to live a lie. And sooner or later the decision may be made for you.

Disadvantages of telling

★ You may get the sack (although legislation may soon be passed affecting this – see below) or not get the job in the first place.

However, if you think telling your boss would result in dismissal, you may be better off looking for another job.
★ Your colleagues may not understand and their fear and ignorance could make matters worse.
★ You may be overlooked for promotion.

Advantages of not telling

★ If you are coping now, and assuming your condition does not change, why make waves?
★ You can find a more suitable job in your own time.
★ You can save money in case things do get worse.

On balance, even though you may come up with more reasons not to tell, you will probably feel better if you *do* tell people at work. Otherwise you may find yourself feeling guilty and even ashamed, which is not good for the self-esteem. However, this very much depends on your own circumstances.

The law
As a result of intensive lobbying from disability organisations, the Government has recently introduced Civil Rights legislation which will help prevent disabled people being discriminated against. It will focus primarily on employment.

When he introduced the bill in late 1994, the then minister for disabled people William Hague said it would become 'unlawful for an employer to treat a disabled person less favourably than he would treat others, unless there are justifiable reasons'. Some commentators, both disabled and non-disabled, have questioned whether the bill will really provide adequate protection. 'William Vague', pronounced one headline.

The specific proposals of the bill are unclear at the time of writing. Whatever happens, it makes sense as a person with arthritis to find out if the Civil Rights Act will do anything for you. If your arthritis affects your work, it should do.

The new law will replace the existing legislation you may have heard of, such as the unenforced quota system, and will be stronger than the current 'protection' offered to people registered with the employment service as disabled.

Practical help at work

Access To Work
Your local high street Job Centre offers a number of services. Most importantly, it can put you in contact with a Disability Employment Adviser (DEA) who will discuss with you your eligibility for the Access To Work scheme. You do not have to be registered as disabled, although the DEA will also advise you of the benefits of registering.

Access To Work seeks to allow people with disabilities to compete in the job market on a more equal footing. It is for anyone – whether working, unemployed or self-employed – who has a disability which affects the type of work they can do and which will last longer than one year.

Under the scheme, specialist support and equipment is made available over five years. The support is for you, not your employer, so it doesn't matter if you change job. Unless any of the adaptations bring wider benefit to the business, your employer pays nothing. It is well worth finding out whether you are eligible – it can make the difference between continuing a career or not.

Most employers do not know about Access To Work. They assume that appointing someone with a disability such as arthritis will be more expensive than employing someone without. It is therefore worth checking what help would be available to you before applying for jobs, so you can inform your potential employer. They can find out about the scheme from the Employment Service leaflet PGP10.

In practice, the Access To Work process can take considerable time. The sooner you find out what you are entitled to the better. For further information consult the Employment Service leaflet PCL8, Access To Work. The leaflet PCL2, Make It Work also includes useful advice for disabled job-seekers.

The Employment Service Disability Symbol
Around one thousand employers particularly keen to employ disabled people display an Employment Service 'two-ticks' symbol, which reads 'positive about disabled people'. These companies make five commitments in order to be authorised to use the symbol, including to interview all disabled applicants meeting the minimum criteria for a job, and to make every effort to ensure that employees who become disabled are able to remain in a job.

Ask your DEA about local 'two-ticks' employers.

Your employment options
We all have different ambitions, different skills and different lifestyles. What suits one person will not suit another. Fortunately, there are a range of employment options for people with arthritis. Depending on what you want and what your arthritis allows, one or more may work for you:

★ regular full-time nine-to-five work
★ more flexible working day or week
★ adapted working environment or special equipment
★ retraining
★ part-time work (check on Social Security benefits – see below)
★ job-sharing a post with a colleague
★ working from home
★ seasonal or temporary work (be careful – this may well have an impact on benefits)
★ studying for further qualifications to help you develop or change your career
★ becoming a volunteer can be a bridge to paid employment as well as valuable in itself
★ self-employment

If you're still unconvinced that people with arthritis have exceptional skills, try this for size:

'Being a financial adviser cum debt collector, combined with long hours and problems at home, soon took its toll. My RA flared. After normal working hours we were expected to repossess items from clients who could no longer continue their payments. My inflammation and pain was at its worst at the end of the day. On this particular occasion I was invited in. After explaining why I was there, I tried to pick up the item in question: a video-recorder. Horror struck, I couldn't. I tried again. The picture flashed through my mind of next day in the office: no video-recorder, black looks. Then an idea came to me. Well, it wouldn't hurt to ask. I looked at my client and said, "Could you possibly carry it out to my car? I'm afraid I can't manage it." Silence. For an age, it seemed, before he replied, "Okay, but I wouldn't do it for anyone else." I could have kissed him!'

SOCIAL SECURITY BENEFITS

Reading our newspapers you could be forgiven for thinking that anyone claiming state benefits is a scrounger or swindler. In fact, quite the opposite is true: many benefits go unclaimed or underclaimed by people who are legally entitled to them. This is particularly true of people with mild to moderate arthritis.

The Government's social security benefits system exists to support people who, from circumstances beyond their control, are unable to support themselves because they either cannot work or earn too little money. If that sounds like you, then claim. It's your right. If in doubt, claim.

Most social security benefits are administered through the Department of Social Security's Benefits Agency (BA). You can pick up claim forms and official information leaflets (the most useful introductions are BG1 A Guide to Benefits and FB2 Which Benefit?) at your local BA, the post office or any advice agency.

Some benefits are contributory (they depend on you having paid national insurance) and some are means-tested, but many are not. Many people with arthritis, for example, are entitled to Disability Living Allowance (DLA), particularly the component paid to help you deal with mobility problems. DLA is not taxable, not means-tested and non-contributory. It can entitle you to other benefits.

Social security benefits rates usually change every year and the system itself seems to change almost as often. Arthritis Care, finances permitting, produce an annual magazine called Benefits for Beginners which outlines benefit entitlement in a straightforward and easy-to-read format. Alternatively, try the Government's Benefits Enquiry Line for disabled people; the Disability Alliance, a voluntary organisation who also have a helpline; your local disability information organisation; or the Citizens' Advice Bureau.

Sources of further information on benefits are listed in Chapter 13.

THE WIDER ENVIRONMENT

Houses, public and commercial buildings, roads and the transport system, leisure facilities: our environment is actually designed for the benefit of a minority. Virtually nothing that would improve the environment for people with arthritis would worsen it for anybody else. In fact most people would benefit – other disabled people, mums with kids, the kids themselves, older people . . .

Of course, home is where the heart is, and getting it right for you is the most important thing. It's your place where you can do as you please. It's a retreat, but don't let it become a fortress. Join with other people in your area to ensure that other local facilities are just as accessible – libraries, cinemas, pubs, buses and trains, everywhere. Find out about your local Arthritis Care group or disabled persons' organisation. You'll be doing yourself and a lot of other people a favour. You can't expect others to understand people with arthritis and other disabilities if they never see people with arthritis. Ending ignorance begins with integration.

OUT AND ABOUT

That is not to say that getting out and about is easy. It seldom is. A good general guide to personal and public transport is *Door To*

Door, published by the Department of Transport. An organisation called Tripscope can help with planning journeys.

Motoring
Many people with arthritis can drive. As with the home, there are many adaptations and aids available to help. Some, such as power-steering and automatic transmission, are now standard on some vehicles. For advice on how to meet more specialist needs (and believe me, they probably can be met), contact the Mobility Advice and Information Service at Crowthorne, or the Banstead Mobility Centre.

People receiving the higher rate of the mobility component of Disability Living Allowance can use it to buy or lease a car from Motability, a government initiative to get disabled people mobile.

There are concessions available to certain disabled motorists, including exemption from road tax, the use of disabled parking bays, and the Orange Badge scheme which allows parking in otherwise restricted areas (such as on yellow lines). There is a leaflet, *The Orange Badge Scheme*, and applications are through local authority social security departments.

Sources of further information are listed in Chapter 13.

Rail travel
Travelling by rail is getting easier. British Rail produce leaflets on their facilities for disabled people including the Disabled Persons Railcard. RADAR produces *A Guide to British Rail for Disabled People* which gives access details to over 500 stations. The future, under privatisation, is less certain.

Bus travel
Contact your local bus company for details of accessible buses. There are also Dial-a-Ride schemes in many areas. Contact your local disability advice organisation.

Holidays
There is not space in a book of this size to go into detail on this subject. The Holiday Care Service or Arthritis Care may be able

to help. If you're interested in travelling further afield, the book *Nothing Ventured*, a collection of articles from disabled travellers that truly covers the world, is inspirational. It was edited by Alison Walsh, who has rheumatoid arthritis.

CHAPTER 12

Your Way Ahead

A friend with arthritis once said to me: 'Life is a journey, not a destination.' This is an incredibly liberating thought. Wherever you are now is simply a place *en route*. It is not, as it can seem when you are first diagnosed with arthritis, the end of the road. Arthritis is not your lot, your destiny – the reality of living with arthritis is just one of the many experiences you will have on your journey. You can still go in any direction you choose.

Take on the arthritis, learn from the challenges it brings and continue along your road. It is not easy – accepting arthritis may be one of the hardest things you'll ever do. It may seem very difficult to move on – it may be uphill for a while – but it's not a race, so take your time.

Mark Doughty is thirty-four and has had rheumatoid arthritis for ten years. Now a disability consultant, the positive message he delivers has inspired many people to take back control of their lives and build their own futures.

'When my arthritis took hold, I saw it as something separate from me – that is fatal. It is only when you start to own it that you can move on. It's not about guilt or blame, but you are your body just as you are your mind, your spirit and your emotions. You are more than these things but you are them.

'My girlfriend at the time said to me, "I can't live with three people. I can't live with you, me and the arthritis." That image has stayed with me.'

Taking arthritis on board does not mean being taken over by it. Be honest with yourself about how it makes you feel physically, but remember that most of the problems it brings are not the result of the disease itself but of attitudes and the environment. Maintain as full a life as possible, including your work, your leisure, your hobbies, your family, your friends, your personal relationships, your spirit, your hopes, your ambitions, your work on yourself and your arthritis.

'You have to find your own pathway,' Mark says. 'It's taken me ten years. You have to get in touch with your body. The relationship between a person and their arthritis is fundamental. I was looking around outside all the time because I didn't trust myself and what I am.

'But disease is exactly that, it's dis-ease. It occurs when you're not happy with yourself. You have to engage with that.'

There is no right way ahead – you have to find your own way and you will. This book has explored some possibilities which you might like to take further. It can be tough and, if it's tough on your own, involve others – other people with arthritis, a counsellor, whoever feels right. 'Find yourself someone who has done what you think you'd like to. Follow your intuition.' It's okay to retrace your steps if a particular route isn't working for you.

For Mark Doughty, 'arthritis has been the most profound life-changing experience that I could have had. It's helped me to grow and change. It's challenged me. It's helped me to grasp life fully, and it's helping me to constantly become a better person.

'The skills you need to develop when you have arthritis are skills everybody else needs but unfortunately usually haven't developed. Disability can provide you with an experience and knowledge that most other people don't have. If you use the wisdom that goes with that, you will become much more of a total human being and have much more chance of finding and fulfilling your potential.

'You can come alive.'

CHAPTER 13

The Arthritis Directory

BIBLIOGRAPHY

The Arthritis Helpbook, Kate Lorig and James Fries (Addison Wesley Publishing, 1990) UK Price £11.95 ISBN 0201524031

Arthritis at Your Age, Jill Holroyd (Grindle Press, 1992) £11.95 ISBN 0951881604

Directory for Disabled People, Ann Darnborough and Derek Kinrade (Prentice Hall with RADAR, published annually) £24.95 ISBN 0134330617

All About Arthritis: Past, Present and Future, Derrick Brewerton (Harvard University Press, 1995) £9.95 ISBN 0674016165

Living with Arthritis, J. Shenkman (F. Watts, 1990) £7.99 ISBN 0749601000

How to Conquer Arthritis, Dr Vernon Coleman (Hamlyn, 1993) £7.99 ISBN 0600575225

The *Coping* Series, Robert H. Phillips (Avery) £8.95. Includes *Coping with Osteoarthritis* (1990) ISBN 0895293935, *Coping with Rheumatoid Arthritis* (1989) ISBN 0895293714, *Coping with Lupus* (1987) ISBN 0895292521

Lupus: A Guide for Patients, G.R.V. Hughes (St Thomas Hospital Lupus Trust) £1.35, available from Arthritis Care, address below

Understanding Osteoporosis, W. Cooper (Arrow, 1990) £3.99, ISBN 0099706202

Back Pain: A Handbook for Sufferers, Loic Burn and John Paterson (Headway, 1993) £4.99 ISBN 0340597623

The Good Doctor Guide, Martin Page (Simon & Schuster, 1993) £9.99 ISBN 0671711652

A–Z of Your Rights Under the NHS and Community Care Legislation, Catherine Grimshaw (MIND Publications, 1993) £2.50 – contact MIND Publications, Granta House, 15–19 Broadway, Stratford, London E15 4BQ (0181 519 2122)

The Community Care Handbook: The Reformed System Explained, Barbara Meredith (Age Concern England, 1995) £12.90 ISBN 0862421713

The Balanced Approach, editor Jim Pollard (Arthritis Care, 1995) free, but donation invited, address below

Complementary Medicine and Disability: Alternatives for People with Disabling Conditions, Andrew Vickers (Chapman and Hall, 1993) £14.99 ISBN 0412486903

Complementary Medicine, British Medical Association (BMA/OUP, 1993) £7.99 – contact BMA Publishing Department, BMA House, Tavistock Square, London WC1H 9JR (0171 387 4499)

Food for Thought, Dr Gail Darlington (Arthritis Care, 1995) free, but donation invited, address below

The Complete Guide to Food Allergy and Intolerance, Dr J. Brostoff and L. Gamlin (Bloomsbury, 1993) £5.99 ISBN 0747515107

Enjoy Healthy Eating, Health Education Authority (1995) free from your GP or local HEA, or 60p from Martsons Book Services (01865 204745)

Talk About Pain, editors Jim Pollard and Penny Boot (Arthritis

Care, 1994), free, but donation invited, address below

Coping Successfully with Pain, Neville Shone (Sheldon, 1995) £6.99 ISBN 0859697509

In Pain? A Self-Help Guide for Chronic Pain Sufferers, Chris Wells and Graham Nown (Optima, 1993) £7.99 ISBN 0356210154

Meditation: A Foundation Course, Barry Long (The Barry Long Foundation, 1986) £4.95 ISBN 1899324003

Simple Relaxation, Laura Mitchell (John Murray, 1987) £6.95 ISBN 0719543886

Stop Counting Sheep: Self Help for Insomnia Sufferers, Paul Clayton (Headline Health Kicks, 1994) £5.99 ISBN 0747243360

Feel the Fear and Do It Anyway: How to Turn Your Fear and Indecision into Confidence and Action, Susan Jeffers (Arrow, 1991) £4.99 ISBN 0099741008

Exercise Beats Arthritis: How to Develop Your Own Personal Exercise Programme, V. Sayce and I. Fraser (Thorsens, 1992) £9.99 ISBN 0722527160

Arthritis: Your Complete Exercise Guide, Neil Gordon, The Cooper Clinic, Dallas (Human Kinetics Publishers, 1993) £8.95 ISBN 0873223926

Aquarobics: Getting Fit and Keeping Fit in the Swimming Pool, Glenda Baum (Arrow, 1991) £9.99 ISBN 0099875101

Rebounding for Health and Fitness, Margaret Hawkins (Thorsons, 1993) £4.99 ISBN 0722528647

Back in Action: Do You Have Backache? This Book Will Put it Right, Sarah Key (Vermilion, 1993) £8.99 ISBN 0091786541

Treat Your Own Neck and *Treat Your Own Back*, both by Robin McKenzie (Spinal Publications, 1992) £7.99 each ISBN 0473002094 and 0959774661

Our Relationships, Our Sexuality, Kata Kolbert (Arthritis Care, 1992) £3.00, or free to Arthritis Care members, address below

Living, Loving and Ageing: Sexual and Personal Relationships in Later Life, W. and S. Greengross (Age Concern, 1989) £4.95 ISBN 0862420709

The Baby Challenge: A Handbook on Pregnancy for Women with a Physical Disability, M.J. Campion (Routledge, 1990) £12.99 ISBN 0415048591

Equipment for Disability: A Guide to Provision, Michael Mandelstam (Disabled Living Foundation, 1991) £2.00 ISBN 0901908541

Equipment and Services for People with Disabilities, Department of Health booklet HB6 (1990) available free from Health Publications Unit, No. 2 Site, Heywood Stores, Manchester Road, Heywood, OL10 2PZ

Arthritis – An Equipment Guide, The Disability Information Trust (1991) £6.25, available from The Disability Information Trust, Mary Marlborough Centre, Nuffield Orthopaedic Centre, Headington, Oxford OX3 7LD (01865 227592)

Choosing a Chair, Disabled Living Foundation (address below) £2.00

Are You Sitting Comfortably?, Arthritis Research Council (address below) free

The Disability Casebook, Hobsons Publishing plc, Bateman Street, Cambridge CB2 1LZ (01223 354551) £7.99 ISBN 1853249386

Benefits for Beginners, Arthritis Care (address below) free, reprinted annually

Nothing Ventured, Alison Walsh (Rough Guides, Harrap Columbus, Penguin, 1991) £7.99 ISBN 0747102082

A Guide to British Rail for Disabled People, RADAR (address below) £4.50

AA Guide for the Disabled Traveller, free to AA members or £3.99 from bookshops, ISBN 0749509724

The Disabled Motorist 1995, RADAR/Disabled Motor Club (address below) £2.50

Guide to Services in the UK offering Advice, Information and Assessment to Disabled and Elderly Motorists (1993) free from Department of Transport Mobility Unit, Great Minster House, 76 Marsham Street, London SW1P 4DR (0171 276 0800)

ADDRESSES

Please enclose SAEs when writing to smaller charities.

Arthritis Care, 18 Stephenson Way, London NW1 2HD (0171 916 1500, freephone helpline 0800 289170 noon–4pm, Mon–Fri) – With 70,000 members and over 650 local groups, Arthritis Care offers information, counselling and self-help courses. Its publications include the quarterly magazine *Arthritis News*. Young Arthritis Care is a special section for the under 45s. Membership costs £5 a year.

Arthritis and Rheumatism Council for Research, Copeman House, St Mary's Court, St Mary's Gate, Chesterfield, S41 7TD (01246 558033, freephone helpline 0500 276413) – The leading research organisation in the UK, the ARC produces booklets and

Getting a Grip

factsheets written by doctors and also a quarterly magazine, *Arthritis Today*.

Arachnoiditis Trust, PO Box 3, North Tawton EX20 2YU (01837 89164)

Arthrogryposis Group (TAG), 1 The Oaks, Gillingham, Dorset SP8 4FW (01747 822655)

Behcet's Syndrome Society, 3 Church Close, Lambourn, Hungerford, Berks RG17 8PU (01488 71116)

British Sjogren's Syndrome Association, Madeline Ford, 20 Kingston Way, Nailsea, Bristol BS19 2RA (01275 854215)

Dermatomyositis & Polymyositis Support Group, 146 Newtown Road, Woolston, Southampton, Hants SO19 9HR (01703 449708)

Ehlers-Danlos Support Group, Mrs Valerie Burrows, 1 Chandler Close, Richmond, North Yorks DL10 5QQ (01748 823867)

Ekbom Support Group (Restless Leg Syndrome), 2 The Green, Chedburgh, Bury St Edmunds, Suffolk IP29 4UE

Fibromyalgia Association (UK), Mrs Barbara Doodson, 8 Rochester Grove, Hazel Grove, Stockport, Cheshire SK7 4JD (0161 483 3155)

Hypermobility Syndrome Association, Ms Jane Butler, 10 Wolfester Terrace, Sparkford, Somerset BA22 7JE (01935 851344)

Kawasaki Syndrome Support Group, Sue Davidson, 13 Norwood Grove, Potters Green, Coventry CV2 2FR (01203 612178)

Lupus UK, 51 North Street, Romford, Essex RM1 1BA (01708 731251)

Marfan Association UK, 6 Queens Road, Farnborough, Hants GU14 6DH (01252 547441)

National Ankylosing Spondylitis Society, 3 Grosvenor Crescent, London SW1X 7ER (0171 235 9585)

National Association for the Relief of Pagets Disease, 207 Eccles Old Road, Salford M6 8HA (0161 707 9225)

National Back Pain Association, The Old Office Block, Elmtree Road, Teddington, Middlesex (0181 977 5475)

National Osteoporosis Society, Rosemary Rowe, PO Box 10, Radstock, Bath BA3 3XB (01761 471771; Helpline: 01761 472721)

Perthes Association, 42 Woodland Road, Guildford GU1 1RW (01483 306637)

Polyarteritis (Vasculitis) Contact, M. Gentle, 15 Chepstow Grove, Rednal, Birmingham B45 8EG

Psoriatic Arthropathy Support Group, 136 High Street, Bushey, Herts WD2 3DJ (01923 672837)

Raynaud's and Scleroderma Association, Anne Mawdsley, 112 Crewe Road, Alsager, Cheshire ST7 2JA (01270 872776)

Reflex Sympatetic Dystrophy Support Line: 01276 858253 (Mon 9am–noon) and 01344 885837 (Thurs 9am–noon)

Relapsing Polychondritis Support Group, c/o Miss C.R. Finnett, 63b Cantelupe Road, Bexhill-on-Sea, East Sussex TN40 1PP (01424 730969)

Repetitive Strain Injury (RSI) Association, Chapel House, 152–156 High Street, Yiewsley, West Drayton, Middlesex UB7 7BE (01895 431134)

Restricted Growth Association, Michael Dawson, PO Box 18, Rugeley, Staffordshire WS15 2GH (01889 576571)

Sarcoidosis Association UK, Mrs Anita Cook, 19 Ashurst Close, off Ashurst Drive, Blackbrook, St Helens, Lancashire WA11 9DN (01744 28020)

Scleroderma Society, Mrs Pamela Webster, 61 Sandpit Lane, St Albans, Herts AL1 4EY (01727 855054)

Scoliosis Association UK, 2 Ivebury Court, 325 Latimer Road, London W10 6RA (0181 964 5343)

Wegeners Granulomatosis Support Group, Mr T. Clay, Hillside, 30 Main Street, Halton Village, Runcorn, Cheshire WA7 2AN (01928 563243)

Young Fibromyalgia and Spondylitis Support Group, Vicky Ibbetson, 49 Wash Lane, Clacton-on-sea, Essex CO15 1UR

OTHER USEFUL ADDRESSES

RADAR, 12 City Forum, 250 City Road, London EC1V 8AF (0171 250 3222)

British Council of Organisations of Disabled People (BCODP), Litchurch Plaza, Litchurch Lane, Derby DE24 8AA (01332 295551)

Disability Information and Advice Lines (DIALs), DIAL UK, Park Lodge, St Catherine's Hospital, Tickhill Road, Doncaster TN4 8QN (01302 310123). Local branches.

The Health Information Service 0800 665544

Chartered Society of Physiotherapy, 14 Bedford Row, London WC1R 4ED (0171 242 1941)

College of Health, St Margaret's House, 21 Old Ford Road, London E2 9PL (0181 983 1225)

British Acupuncture Council, Park House, 206 Latimer Road, London W10 2RE (0181 964 0222)

The Shiatsu Society, 5 Foxcote, Wokingham, Berkshire RG40 3PG (01734 730836)

The Society of Teachers of the Alexander Technique, 20 London House, 266 Fulham Road, London SW10 9EL (0171 351 0828)

The British Chiropractic Association, 29 Whitley Street, Reading, Berks RG2 0EG (01734 757557)

The Society for the Promotion of Nutritional Therapy, PO Box 47, Heathfield, East Sussex TN21 8ZX (01435 867007)

The National Institute of Medical Herbalists, 56 Longbrook Street, Exeter, Devon EX4 6AH (01392 426022)

The Society of Homeopaths [for non-medical homeopaths], 2 Artizan Road, Northampton NN1 4HU (01604 21400)

The British Homeopathic Association [for medical homeopaths] 27a Devonshire Street, London W1N 1RJ (0171 935 2163)

The Institute for Complementary Medicine, PO Box 194, London SE16 1QZ (0171 237 5165)

The General Council and Register of Osteopaths, 56 London Street, Reading, Berkshire RG1 4SQ (01734 576585)

Association of Reflexologists, 27 Old Gloucester Street, London WC1N 3XX (01892 512612)

The British Association for Counselling, 1 Regent Place, Rugby CV21 2PJ (01788 578328)

Pain-Wise UK, 33 Kingsdown Park, Tankerton, Kent CT5 2DT (01227 277886)

Pain Concern UK, PO Box 318, Canterbury CT4 5DP (telephone helpline 01227 264677 Mon–Fri 10am–4pm)

Pain Relief Foundation, Rice Lane, Liverpool L9 1AE (0151 523 1486)

SPOD (Association to aid the personal and sexual relationships of people with disabilities), 286 Camden Road, London N7 0BJ (0171 607 8851)

Disabled Living Centres Council, 1st Floor, Winchester House, 11 Cranmer Road, London SW9 6EJ (0171 820 0567)

Disabled Living Foundation (DLF), 380–84 Harrow Road, London W9 2HU (0171 289 6111)

Department of the Environment, 2 Marsham Street, London SW1 (0171 276 0900) – produces various publications for people requiring adaptations to their living quarters

Age Concern, Astral House, 1268 London Road, London SW16 4ER (0181 679 8000)

Opportunities for People with Disabilities, 1 Bank Buildings, Princes Street, London EC2R 8EU (0171 726 4961)

Computability Centre, PO Box 94, Warwick, Warwickshire CV34 5WS (01926 312847, freephone advice line 0800 269545)

The Arthritis Directory

Association of Disabled Professionals, 170 Benton Hill, Wakefield Road, Horbury, West Yorkshire WF4 5HW (01924 270335)

Skill: National Bureau for Students with Disabilities, 336 Brixton Road, London SW9 7AA (information service 0171 978 9890, Mon–Fri 1.30–4.30pm)

Benefits Agency (leaflets BG1 *A Guide to Benefits*, FB2 *Which Benefit*), BA Distribution and Storage Centre, Manchester Road, Heywood, Lancashire OL10 2PZ

The Benefits Enquiry Line for People with Disabilities, 8th Floor, Victoria House, Ormskirk Road, Preston, PR1 2QP (freephone 0800 882200 for advice or 0800 441144 for help with completing claim forms)

Disability Alliance, 88–94 Wentworth Street, London E1 7SA (rights advice line 0171 247 8763 Mondays and Wednesdays 2–4pm)

Banstead Mobility Centre, Fountain Drive, Carshalton, Surrey SM5 4NR (0181 770 1151)

MAVIS (Mobility Advice and Vehicle Information Service), TRL, Old Wokingham Road, Crowthorne, Berks RG45 6AU (01344 770456)

Disabled Drivers Association, National Headquarters, Ashwellthorpe, Norwich, NR16 1EX (01508 489449)

Disabled Drivers Motor Club, Cottingham Way, Thrapston, Northants NN14 4PL (01832 734724)

Motability, 2nd Floor, Gate House, West Gate, Harlow, Essex CM20 1HR (01279 635666)

Index

Access To Work scheme 155
acupuncture 69–70
   see also shiatsu, TENS machines
adapting house to needs 147–8
adverse neural tension stretches 30
aerobic exercise 124–5
aids for everyday tasks 139, 141–7, 159
alcohol 19, 55, 58, 59, 93
Alexander Technique 72–4
alternative medicine see complementary therapy
analgesics 54–5
ankylosing spondylitis 11–12, 23–4, 101
anti-malarial drugs 58
Aquarobics 127
aromatherapy 27, 81–3
arthritis 2, 5
   causes 6, 24
   hereditary factors 23–4
   in children 16–17
   treatment see treatment of arthritis
arthritis, attitudes to 1–2, 28, 106, 131–8
   and being gay/lesbian 138
   and building self-esteem 133–4
   and communication 134–5
   and love-making 135–8
   charities' image of arthritis 132–3
   employers' 29, 149–53
   media images of arthritis 132–3
   medical profession 2, 8, 17–18, 30, 32–3, 114
   of people with arthritis 103–5
arthritis, categories 6–7
   crystals 7
   degenerative 7
   infective 7
   inflammatory 6
   muscular 7
   periarticular 7
arthritis, forms 7–9, 11–16
   see also back pain
   ankylosing spondylitis 11–12, 23–4
   gout 12–13
   Juvenile Chronic Arthritis 16–17
   lumbar spondylosis 11
   osteoarthritis 7–8, 11, 19
   psoriatic 15–16, 23–4
   psoriatic arthropathy 16
   reactive 14–15, 23–4
   Reiter's Disease 15
   repetitive strain injury (RSI) 20–22, 29–31
   rheumatoid 8–9, 23–4
   systemic lupus erythematosus 13–14, 23
   work-related 20–22, 29–31
arthritis, psychological aspect 3–4, 31, 34–6, 103–20
   and pain 110–17
   counselling 117–18
   meditation 116–17
   personal development 118–19
   positive thinking 106
   psychotherapy 117–18
   relaxation 115–16
   self-help 107–10
      groups 119–20

self-image 106–7
self-management 107–10
stress 114–15
arthritis, symptoms 1
  ankylosing spondylitis 11–12
  gout 12
  Juvenile Chronic Arthritis 16–17
  lumbar spondylosis 11
  osteoarthritis 7–8, 11
  psoriatic 16
  psoriatic arthropathy 16
  reactive 14–15
  Reiter's Disease 15
  repetitive strain injury (RSI) 22
  rheumatoid 9
  systemic lupus erythematosus 13–14
  work-related 22
Arthritis and Rheumatism Council 109
Arthritis At Your Age (Holroyd) 48
Arthritis Care (organisation) 27, 44, 109–10

back pain 10–11
  see also arthritis (forms)
  lower 11
  neck 10–11
  spine 10
bathrooms 144
beds 145
benefits, social security 157–8
blood cells 40–41
blood tests 40–41
bones 18–20
bowel infection 14
buses and disability 159

calcium 18, 101–2
carbohydrates 95
carpal tunnel syndrome 22
causes of arthritis *see* arthritis, causes
chairs 144–5
charities' image of arthritis 132–3
children, arthritis in 16–17
chiropractic 74–5
  see also osteopathy
cholesterol 92, 124
  see also fat
choosing complementary therapies 68–9

clinics, pain 113–14
clothing 148–9
cod-liver oil 97
cold in combatting pain 113
communication and attitudes 134–5
Community Care 45–6, 147
  see also treatment
complementary therapy 65–88
  acupuncture 69–70
  Alexander Technique 72–4
  and placebo effect 66–7
  and power principle 67
  aromatherapy 81–3
  chiropractic 74–5
  choosing 68–9
  herbal medicine 76–8
  homeopathy 78–81
  massage 81–3
  moxibustion 70
  osteopathy 84–5
  practitioners 65–6, 68–9
  reflexology 85–6
  shiatsu 71–2
  Tai-chi 88
  TENS (transcutaneous electrical nerve stimulation) machines 71
  yoga 87–8
computer keyboards and RSI 21
computers, voice-operated 30–31, 139
  see also word-processors
concentrative meditation 117
consultants, hospital 38–41
  referral to 38–9
cooking 142–4
counselling 117–18
  see also psychotherapy
crystals (arthritis) 7
cures, research into 109
cycling 127–8
  see also static cycling

degenerative arthritis 7
diet 33, 89–102
  see also dietary supplements, weight
  alcohol 93
  and ankylosing spondylitis 101
  and gout 12–13, 102
  and osteoarthritis 101
  and osteoporosis 101–2

Index

and systemic lupus erythematosus 101
cholesterol 92
fat 91–2, 95–6
fibre 90–91, 96
food labels 95–6
healthy eating, guide to 90
manipulation 97–100
minerals 92–3
salt 93, 96
starch 90–91
sugar 93
vitamins 92–3
dietary supplements 97–8
see also diet
Evening Primrose oil 97–8
fish oils 97, 101
garlic 98
iron 98
New Zealand Green-Lipped Mussel 98
selenium 98
disability 104–5
and transport 158–60
discrimination, legislation against 154–5
Disability Living Allowance 157, 159
DMARDs (disease-modifying anti-rheumatic drugs) 56–8
drugs 51–64
see also treatment
analgesics 54–5, 111–12
and immune system 53–4
anti-malarial 58
categories 52–3
DMARDs 56–8
immunosuppressors 58–9
industry 52–3
maximising effects of 61–4
narcotics 54–5
NSAIDs 55–6
painkillers 54–5
research 52–3
side-effects 51, 54–61, 64
steroids 59–61

electricity 145
employers, attitudes of 149–53

employment
financial help for 30–31
options 156
endurance exercise 124
cycling 127–8
see also static cycling
swimming 125–6
see also hydrotherapy
walking 125
energy (in food) 95
environment factors in RSI 22
epicondylitis 22
essential oils 81–3
Evening Primrose oil 97–8
exclusion diets *see* diet, manipulation
exercise 19, 28, 30, 121–9
aerobic 124–5
cycling 127–8
endurance 124–9
gymnasium equipment 129
programmes 121–2
pulse rate 122
range of movement 123
sport 129
static cycling 128
strengthening 123–4
stretching 123
swimming 125–6
see also hydrotherapy
walking 125
extending aids 145–6

fastenings, clothing 148
fat 91–2, 95–6
see also cholesterol
Feel The Fear And Do It Anyway (Jeffers) 108
fertility 59
fibre 90–91, 96
fibromyalgia 18
fibrositis 17
financial help for employment 30–31
fish oils 97, 101
focused breathing (meditation) 117
food labels 95–6

garlic 98
gas 145

gay people with arthritis, attitudes to 138
general practitioners (GPs) 37–9, 46–9
  see also medical profession (attitudes)
Good Doctor Guide, The 44
gout 12–13, 102
GPs see general practitioners
gripping/grabbing aids 145–6
gymnasium equipment 129

haematology see blood tests
health professionals 37–49
  see also medical profession (attitudes)
  consultants, hospital 38–41
  general practitioners (GPs) 37–9, 46–9
  occupational therapists 42–3
  patient's relationship with 46–9, 67–8
  physiotherapists 41–2
  rheumatologists see consultants
  surgeons 43–5
healthy eating, guide to 90
heat in combatting pain 112–13
height–weight chart 94
herbal medicine 76–8
hereditary factors in arthritis 23–4
hip replacement 43
HLA B27 (cell group) 15, 23–4
holidays 159–60
home, managing arthritis in see managing arthritis at home
homeopathy 78–81
Hormone Replacement Therapy (HRT) 19
hospital consultants see consultants
house, adapting 147–8
housework 146–7
HRT (Hormone Replacement Therapy) 19
hydrotherapy 27, 42
  see also swimming

ideal weight 94–5
immune system 9, 13, 20, 41, 53–4
immunosuppressors 58–9

infection 14–15
  of the bowel 14
  sexually transmitted 14-15, 24
infective arthritis 7
inflammatory arthritis 6
iron 98

joints 5–6, 43
Juvenile Chronic Arthritis 16–17
  pauci-articular 16–17
  poly-articular 16
  systemic 16

kitchens 142–4

lesbians with arthritis, attitudes to 138
Lorig, Kate 110
love-making and arthritis 135–8
  lubricants 136
  positions 136–7
lower-back pain 11
lubricants, love-making 136
lumbar spondylosis 11

managing arthritis at home 139–49
  see also managing arthritis at work
  adapting house 147–8
  aids for everyday tasks 139, 141–7
  bathrooms 144
  beds 145
  chairs 144–5
  clothing 148–9
  cooking 142–4
  electricity 145
  fastenings, clothing 148
  gas 145
  help at home 147
  housework 146–7
  kitchens 142–4
  plugs, electric 144
  shoes 148
  sockets, electric 144
  telephones 145
  utilities 145
managing arthritis at work 139–42, 149–57
  see also managing arthritis at home, RSI
  Access To Work scheme 155

Index

attitudes of employers 149–53
discrimination, legislation against 154–5
employment options 156
Employment Service disability symbol 156
recruitment 149–51
self-employment 151
voluntary work 152
manipulation, dietary 97–100
mantra meditation 117
massage 81–3, 112
maximising effects of drugs 61–4
media images of arthritis 132–3
Medical Directory, The 44
medical profession, attitudes 2, 8, 17–18, 30, 32–3, 114
  see also GPs, health professionals
medicines see drugs
meditation 116–17
  see also relaxation
men, ideal weight 95
menopause 18–19
mind, arthritis and see arthritis (psychological aspect)
minerals 92–3
motoring and disability 159
moxibustion 70
muscular diseases 5, 7, 17–18
  fibromyalgia 18
  fibrositis 17
  polymyalgia rheumatica 17

narcotics 54–5
National Health Service (NHS) 30, 80
neck pain 10–11
New Zealand Green-Lipped Mussel 98
NHS (National Health Service) 30, 80
NHS and Community Care Act (1993) 45–6
NSAIDs (non-steroidal anti-inflammatory drugs) 55–6

occupational therapists 42–3
oestrogen 19
oils, fish 97, 101
operations 43–5
osteoarthritis 7–8, 11, 19, 26–8, 101, 123

osteopathy 84–5
  see also chiropractic
osteoporosis 18–20, 101–2
other people, attitudes to arthritis 131–8
Our Relationships, Our Sexuality (Boot) 131, 137

pain 48
  back 10–11
  cold in combatting 113
  drugs in combatting 111–12
  heat in combatting 112–13
  massage in combatting 112
  sex in combatting 113
  sleep in combatting 113
pain, psychological aspect 110–17
  and meditation 116–17
  and relaxation 115–16
  and stress 114–15
  clinics 113–14
  pain gate theory 111–14
painkillers 54–5
Patient's Charter 38, 39, 44, 49
pauci-articular Juvenile Chronic Arthritis 16–17
performing tasks 140–41
periarticular arthritis 7
peritendinitis 22
personal development 118–19
physiotherapy 41–2
placebo effect in complementary therapy 66–7
platelets (blood cells) 41
plugs, electric 144
poly-articular Juvenile Chronic Arthritis 16
polymyalgia rheumatica 17
positive thinking 106
power principle in complementary therapy 67
practitioners (complementary therapy) 65–6, 68–9
prescriptions 64
private treatment 30, 42
problem solving 140–42
programmes, exercise 121–2
prostaglandins 55
psoriasis 15–16

psoriatic arthritis 15–16, 23–4
psoriatic arthropathy 16
psychological aspect of arthritis *see* arthritis (psychological aspect)
psychotherapy 117–18
  see also counselling
pulse rate 122

rail travel and disability 159
range of movement exercises 123
reactive arthritis 14–15, 23–4
recruitment (work) 149–51
red blood cells 41
referral to a consultants 38–9
reflexology 85–6
Reiter's Disease 15
relationships and arthritis 28, 33–4
relationship with health professionals, patient's 46–9, 67–8
relaxation 115–16
  see also meditation
repetitive strain injury (RSI) 20–22, 29–31
  see also managing arthritis at work
  and computer keyboards 21
  carpal tunnel syndrome 22
  causes 22
  epicondylitis 22
  peritendinitis 22
  tendinitis 22
  tenosyvitis 22
research, medical 52–3, 109
rheumatism 5
rheumatoid arthritis 8–9, 23–4, 32–4, 123
  and dietary manipulation 98–100
rheumatoid factor 24
rheumatologists *see* consultants
RSI *see* repetitive strain injury

salt 93, 96
saturated fats 91
selenium 98
self-employment 151
self-esteem 133–4
self-help 107–10
  groups 119–20
self-image 106–7
self-management 107–10

sex in combatting pain 113
sexually transmitted diseases 14-15
sexually transmitted infection 14–15, 24
shiatsu 71–2
  see also acupuncture, TENS machines
shoes 148
side-effects, drugs 51, 64
  analgesics 54–5
  anti-malarial drugs 58
  DMARDs 57–8
  immunosuppressors 59
  narcotics 55
  NSAIDs 55–6
  steroids 60–61
Sjogren's syndrome 20
skin tests 100
sleep in combatting pain 113
social security benefits 157–8
Social Services 45–6
sockets, electric 144
sodium 96
spine 10, 74
sport 129
starch 90–91
static cycling 128
  see also cycling
steroids 18–19
strengthening exercises 123–4
stress 114–15
stretching exercises 123
sugar 93
supplements, dietary *see* dietary supplements
support groups 119–20
surgeons 43–5
swimming 125–6
  see also hydrotherapy
symptoms
  arthritis *see* arthritis (symptoms)
  fibromyalgia 18
  fibrositis 17
  infection 14-15
  Polymyalgia Rheumatica 17
  psoriasis 15
  Sjogren's syndrome 20
systemic Juvenile Chronic Arthritis 16

Index

systemic lupus erythematosus 13–14, 23, 101

tablets (steroids) 60
Tai-Chi 88
telephones 145
tendinitis 22, 29–31
tenosyvitis 22
TENS (transcutaneous electrical nerve stimulation) 71
TENS machines 71
  see also acupuncture, shiatsu
tests 40–41, 100
trans-fats 91
transport and disability 158–60
treatment of arthritis
  see also drugs, Community Care
  NHS 30, 37–45, 46–9
  private 30, 42
tumour necrosis factor 54

ulcers, peptic 27, 56
unsaturated fats 91
uric acid 12
utilities 145

visualisation (meditation) 116–17
vitamin D 18–19
vitamins 92–3
voice-recognition computers 30–31, 139
  see also word-processors
voluntary work 152

walking 125
weight 93–5
  see also diet
  cutting calories 94
  height–weight chart 94
  ideal 94–5
white blood cells 41
women, ideal weight 94
word-processors 141
  see also computers
work, managing arthritis at see managing arthritis at work
work-related arthritis 20–22, 29–31
work-related upper-limb disorders see RSI

yoga 87–8
Young Arthritis Care 17, 118–20

Headline Health Kicks

THE PRIME OF YOUR LIFE		
Self help during menopause	Pamela Armstrong	£5.99 ☐
STOP COUNTING SHEEP		
Self help for insomnia sufferers	Dr Paul Clayton	£5.99 ☐
AM I A MONSTER, OR IS THIS PMS?		
Self help for PMS sufferers	Louise Rhoddon	£4.99 ☐
GET UP AND GO!		
Self help for fatigue sufferers	Anne Woodham	£5.99 ☐

You can kick that problem!

All Headline books are available at your local bookshop or newsagent, or can be ordered direct from the publisher. Just tick the titles you want and fill in the form below. Prices and availability subject to change without notice.

Headline Book Publishing, Cash Sales Department, Bookpoint, 39 Milton Park, Abingdon, OXON, OX14 4TD, UK. If you have a credit card you may order by telephone – 01235 400400.

Please enclose a cheque or postal order made payable to Bookpoint Ltd to the value of the cover price and allow the following for postage and packing:

UK & BFPO: £1.00 for the first book, 50p for the second book and 30p for each additional book ordered up to a maximum charge of £3.00.

OVERSEAS & EIRE: £2.00 for the first book, £1.00 for the second book and 50p for each additional book.

Name ....

Address ....

....

....

If you would prefer to pay by credit card, please complete:
Please debit my Visa/Access/Diner's Card/American Express (delete as applicable) card no:

Signature .... Expiry Date ....